A clinical guide to general medicine and surgery for dental practitioners
2nd edition

M Greenwood MDS PhD, FDSRCS, MBChB, FRCS, FRCS(OMFS), FHEA
Honorary Clinical Professor and Consultant
Department of Oral and Maxillofacial Surgery
School of Dental Sciences, Newcastle upon Tyne

J G Meechan, BSc, BDS, PhD, FDSRCPS, FDSRCS(Ed)
Senior Lecturer and Honorary Consultant
Department of Oral and Maxillofacial Surgery
School of Dental Sciences, Newcastle upon Tyne

2010
Published by the British Dental Association
64 Wimpole Street, London, W1G 8YS

ACKNOWLEDGEMENTS

The authors are grateful to Dr M. Rudralingam, Consultant in Oral Medicine, University Dental Hospital of Manchester; Dr I. Macleod, Consultant in Dental Radiology, Newcastle Dental Hospital; Dr S. J. Brown, Specialist Registrar in Psychiatry at Newcastle Upon Tyne. Special thanks also to Professor J. V. Soames, Professor R. R. Welbury and Dr U. J. Moore for providing some of the clinical photographs.

ISBN: 978-1-907923-01-2

Printed and bound by Martins The Printers, Berwick upon Tweed.

CONTENTS

Chapter 1
The cardiovascular system

M. Greenwood and J. G. Meechan

IN BRIEF

- Cardiovascular disease is common
- Pain and anxiety increase cardiac load and increase the risk of precipitating angina/arrhythmias
- A thorough history will usually elicit the fact that the patient has cardiovascular disease (summarised in *Table 2*)
- Examination of the patient may reveal cardiovascular disease – cyanosis (central/peripheral), shortage of breath, abnormalities in the pulse, finger clubbing, splinter haemorrhages or ankle oedema
- Drugs used in the treatment of cardiovascular disease impact on patient management.

This book examines aspects of general medicine and surgery which are of relevance to dental practice. The approach is standardised by considering systems under common headings eg history, examination, commonly prescribed drugs and aspects relating to general and local anaesthesia and management in the dental surgery. The first chapter considers the cardiovascular system.

INTRODUCTION

Cardiovascular disease is common and it is inevitable that any practitioner dealing with patients will encounter it. In 1984 it was estimated that 2% of all adult dental patients were receiving anti-hypertensive therapy.[1,2] This figure has risen and in 1997 it was reported that up to 13% of patients in a dental hospital setting and 5% of those attending dental practice were receiving anti-hypertensive drugs.[3] There may be a well-established previous history of cardiovascular disease. The incidence increases with age such that, by the age of 70, all patients will have some degree of cardiovascular disease (this may be very minor and subclinical or the origin not recognised by the patient eg calf claudication, a sign of peripheral vascular disease).

Risk factors for cardiovascular disease are shown in *Table 1*.

In the history it is clearly important to assess the degree of compensation that the patient has managed to achieve, ie how badly the patient is affected by their condition in terms of signs, symptoms and activity. The efficacy of medication is also important. Some patients may be taking aspirin on a regular basis. Specific enquiry is important due to aspirin's effects on blood clotting.

RELEVANT POINTS IN THE HISTORY

Other points to ask in the history (*Table 2*) include the following:

Chest pain

The purpose of questioning here is not to try to be diagnostic but to gain an idea as to whether a cardiovascular cause for the pain may be likely, since some patients may be unaware of their condition but nevertheless be at risk. Features which make the pain unlikely to be cardiac in origin are: pains lasting less that 30 seconds however severe, stabbing pains, well-localised left submammary (under the breast) pain, and pains which continually vary in location. A chest pain made better by stopping exercise is more likely to be cardiac in origin than one that is not related (see Myocardial Infarction, Angina). Pleuritic pain is sharp and made worse on inspiration, eg in pulmonary embolism. Shingles (Varicella Zoster) may cause pain following a particular nerve territory. The characteristic rash is preceded by an area of hyperaesthesia.

Oesophagitis may cause a retrosternal pain which is worse on bending or lying down. However, oesophageal pain, like cardiac pain, may be relieved by sublingual nitrates, eg glyceryl trinitrate (GTN).

Hyperventilation may produce chest pain. Gallbladder and pancreatic disease may also mimic cardiac pain. Musculoskeletal pain is often accompanied by tenderness to palpation in the affected region.

GENERAL MEDICINE AND SURGERY FOR DENTAL PRACTITIONERS

1. The cardiovascular system
2. The respiratory system
3. The gastrointestinal system
4. Neurological disorders
5. Liver disease
6. The endocrine system
7. Renal disorders
8. The musculoskeletal system
9. Haematology and patients with bleeding problems
10. The paediatric patient
11. The older patient
12. Metabolic disorders
13. Skin disorders (A)
14. Skin disorders (B)
15. Psychiatry
16. Cancer, radiotherapy and chemotherapy

Table 1 Risk Factors for Cardiovascular Disease

- Smoking
- Excess alcohol
- Diabetes mellitus
- Hypercholesterolaemia
- Family history of cardiovascular disease
- Sedentary lifestyle
- Obesity

Angina pectoris

This central, crushing chest pain may radiate to the neck, mandible and one or both arms. It may be felt in only one of these sites. Unstable angina is that occurring at rest, minimal exertion or with rapidly increasing severity. There is a significant risk of myocardial infarction and elective surgery should not be carried out on the patient with unstable angina. When performing emergency treatment on such patients the use of epinephrine (adrenaline) containing local anaesthetics is best avoided.[4] The severity of angina may be gauged by the exertion required to provoke an attack, and the efficacy of medication to induce relief.

Effective analgesia, short appointments, availability of oxygen and GTN are all important in treatment regimens. The use of sedation should be considered in these patients as an added stress reduction measure. GTN should relieve chest pain in angina within 5 minutes. A spray formulation is now commonly used; this is the preferred formulation as the emergency medicament in practice as it has a longer shelf-life than the tablet formulation (once the bottle is opened).

Myocardial infarction (MI)

The signs and symptoms of MI are well known and may be like angina but more severe and of longer duration. Importantly, it is not relieved by GTN. Some myocardial infarctions are 'silent', ie occur with no recognised symptoms or signs at the time. The residual deficit is a marker of severity of the original event. Admission to hospital, the coronary care unit and duration of admission are also indicative.

The timings for dental treatment, for both local and general anaesthesia post MI, are given later, but in all cases obviously local analgesia must be maximally effective, and GA carried out in a hospital environment. As mentioned above sedation should be considered for many of these patients.

Hypertension

There is variation but, in general terms, treatment is carried out if the blood pressure is persistently more than 200 Systolic or over 110 Diastolic. Treatment may be indicated at lower levels if vascular complications are evident.

Most hypertension is 'essential' (90%), ie no cause found. The aim of treatment is to maintain a blood pressure less than 160/90. Stress may further increase an already raised blood pressure, leading to risk of stroke or cardiac arrest.

Postural hypotension, eg on suddenly rising from the supine position or rapid alteration of the dental chair, may be a side effect of some antihypertensive drugs. There may be underlying cardiac or renal disease in some patients with hypertension. Many antihypertensive drugs impact on dental management (see later).

Syncope or fainting

This, as is well known, may be precipitated by fear and may be vasovagal or cardiac in origin. Respiratory syncope (in cases of extreme coughing bouts) also exists.

In the 'carotid sinus syndrome', mild pressure on the neck causes syncope with bradycardia or cardiac arrest.

Shortage of breath (SOB)/exercise tolerance

SOB is often a sign of cardiac failure, but must be differentiated from respiratory disease with which, of course, it may co-exist.

The degree of severity can be assessed by enquiring about whether the patient ever wakes up in the night with breathlessness (paroxysmal nocturnal dyspnoea), or has orthopnoea, ie becoming breathless on lying flat at night. The degree of exertion needed to precipitate breathlessness is also important.

In uncontrolled cardiac failure, dental treatment under any form of anaesthesia should be deferred until medication and symptoms are stabilised. Even when relatively well-controlled, putting the patient in the

Table 2 Relevant points in the history with reference to cardiovascular system

- Chest pain
- Angina
- Myocardial infarction
- Hypertension
- Medication eg aspirin, warfarin
- Syncope
- Shortage of breath/exercise tolerance
- Cardiac rate/rhythm
- Cardiomyopathy
- Coronary artery bypass graft
- Valve replacements
- Congenital disorders
- Cardiac transplants
- Rheumatic fever
- Infective endocarditis
- Venous/lymphatic disorders

supine position may exacerbate dyspnoea and is therefore best avoided. Cor Pulmonale is the term used to describe heart failure secondary to he

In 'left-sided heart failure', the oedema is pulmonary, whereas in 'right-sided heart failure' it is peripheral (sacral in the bed-bound and ankles in the ambulant).

Rheumatic Fever

There may not be any subsequent cardiac damage, but this can only be determined definitively by a cardiologist. These patients may be more at risk of life-threatening reactions to prophylactic antibiotics compared with the development of infective endocarditis (see later).[5] A typical rash in a patient allergic to penicillin who has taken the antibiotic is shown in *Fig. 1*.

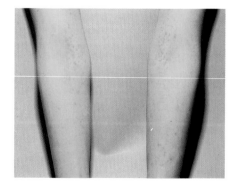

Fig. 1 A typical rash on the forearms of a patient who was given oral penicillin for prophylaxis against infective endocarditis. This is no longer required (see later).

Table 3 Common arrhythmias which may be encountered in dental practice
• Sinus Tachycardia - pulse over 100 beats per minute
• Sinus Bradycardia - pulse less than 60 beats per minute
• Atrial Fibrillation - totally irregular wrist pulse
• Ventricular Extrasystole – 'missed beats' at the wrist

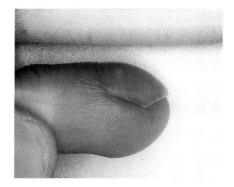

Fig. 2 Finger clubbing. This patient also demonstrates peripheral cyanosis.

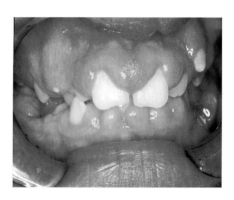

Fig. 3 Gingival hyperplasia in a post-cardiac transplant patient who is taking the calcium channel blocker nifedipine.

COMMON ARRHYTHMIAS (SEE TABLE 3)

Sinus tachycardia (the pulse is more than 100 beats per minute)

This may be physiological (exercise, emotion, anxiety, pain) or be related to fever, post myocardial infarction, shock, heart failure and with some drugs (epinephrine, atropine). Hyperthyroidism, smoking and excessive coffee ingestion may also be causes.

Sinus bradycardia (the pulse is less than 60 beats per minute)

This may occur physiologically in athletes or in vasovagal attack. Drugs such as beta blockers or digoxin may cause it. Post myocardial infarction and the 'sick sinus syndrome' may all be causative, as may hypothyroidism.

Atrial fibrillation

This is common in the elderly and may be asymptomatic. An irregularly irregular pulse is palpable at the wrist. If a wrist pulse is palpated eg after a faint or during sedation, it will frequently be encountered as a pre-existing anomaly.

Ventricular extrasystole

This is the commonest arrhythmia after a myocardial infarction. Three successive extrasystoles are described as ventricular tachycardia. An extra-systole is an 'extra' ventricular contraction. A ventricular extrasystole may be felt as a "missed beat" at the wrist. They are usually of no significance.

Arrhythmias are relevant since they may be exacerbated by dental treatment due to the associated stress, or by general anaesthesia.[8] Common arrhythmias are summarised in *Table 3*. Arrhythmias may be increased by manipulation of eyes, carotid sinus

Table 4 Congenital cardiac defects may be broadly divided into cyanotic and acyanotic categories	
Cyanotic	Acyanotic
Transposition of great vessels	Ventricular septal defect
Fallot's tetralogy - (Ventricular septal defect	Atrial septal defect
Pulmonary stenosis	Patent ductus arteriosus
Right ventricular hypertrophy	Aortic coarctation
Overriding aorta)	

or neck by pathways mediated by the vagus nerve.

Cardiomyopathy

This is a general term meaning disease of the heart muscle. Consultation with the patient's cardiologist is important, particularly where there are associated cardiac symptoms.

Coronary artery bypass graft

Exercise tolerance and history of chest pain should be enquired about post-bypass.

Table 5 The swollen limb - many causes in addition to purely cardiovascular

Systemic Causes
Congestive cardiac failure
Right heart' failure
Hypoalbuminaemia eg nephrotic syndrome
Fluid overload
Regional Causes
Venous obstruction eg advanced pregnancy
Lymphatic obstruction
Local
Sluggish venous return eg poor muscle pump in a paraplegic patient
Acute obstruction to venous return eg DVT, Previous DVT
Cellulitis, lymphatic aplasia/obstruction

Valve replacement

Artificial valves may be tissue or mechanical. The latter patients are placed on life-long warfarin.

Congenital cardiac defects

Congenital cardiac defects may be divided into cyanotic or acyanotic types. In the former, chronic hypoxaemia leads to finger clubbing (Fig. 2) and polycythaemia. The polycythaemia may lead to a tendency to haemolysis or thrombosis. The disorders fitting into the broad categories are shown in Table 4.

Cerebral abscess and bleeding tendency are risks in these patients.

Cardiac transplants

Pre-operatively, it is important to eradicate potential or actual sources of infection and to optimise oral hygiene. Such patients will usually be treated in the hospital setting. Post-transplant treatment may be complicated by:
• Immunosuppression
• Steroid Therapy
• Gingival overgrowth as a result of post-transplant drug therapy[9] (Fig. 3)
• Supersensitivity of the transplanted heart to circulating

catecholamines[10] which may include epinephrine in dental local anaesthetics[11]
• Hepatitis, HIV infection (rarely).

Venous/lymphatic disorders

A swollen limb may be a sign of heart failure. Causes of a swollen limb may be divided into systemic, regional and local as shown in Table 5. For dental purposes, the patient should be treated with legs elevated to minimise dependent oedema, but the practitioner should beware of orthopnoea.

EXAMINATION

The most obvious initial observations are those of the patient's general demeanour, colour, whether short of breath at rest (SOBAR), or on minimal exertion, eg walking into the surgery (obviously primary respiratory causes may also exist). SOBAR indicates severe cardiorespiratory disease. A pulse oximeter reading is a useful rough guide to the efficiency of ventilation.

Cyanosis may be central, eg lip, tongue, or peripheral, eg nail beds (Fig. 2). Cyanosis represents a concentration of desaturated haemoglobin of at least 5 grams per decilitre. The pulse in terms of rate, volume, rhythm and character can give important clues to the state of the cardiovascular system and, indeed, other systems.

Clubbing of the fingers (loss of the angle between nail and nail bed when a finger is viewed from the side) may occur in infective endocarditis, cyanotic congenital heart disease and thyrotoxicosis (in which atrial fibrillation may also be noted).

Splinter haemorrhages are vasculitic consequences of infective endocarditis visible in the nail beds. Osler's Nodes may also occur (painful lesions on the finger pulps) and macules on the palms (Janeway Lesions) in infective endocarditis.

Swollen ankles may be a sign of cardiac failure and oedema occurs in the sacrum in bedbound patients.

DRUGS USED IN CARDIOVASCULAR DISEASE

Beta blockers

These drugs decrease the sympathetic effects on the cardiovascular system, eg atenolol, propranolol, sotalol. Beta-blockade inhibits any reduction in diastolic blood pressure produced by epinephrine in dental local anaesthetics[12] which might result in an uncompensated rise in systolic blood pressure. Thus dose limitation of epinephrine is wise when patients are taking beta blockers, two cartridges of an epinephrine containing solution in an adult is a sensible limit.

Oral side-effects can include dry mouth and lichenoid reactions.

Diuretics

These may be used in hypertension (thiazides only) and heart failure. Patients receiving non potassium sparing diuretics have been shown to experience an increased hypokalaemic response to epinephrine in dental local anaesthetics compared to healthy patients[13] and this could predispose to arrhythmias. A limit of one to two epinephrine containing LA cartridges is recommended.

Digoxin

This is used to slow the ventricular rate in fast atrial fibrillation. The old-fashioned use is in the treatment of heart failure - Angiotensin Converting Enzyme (ACE) Inhibitors are now more commonly used (see below).

Vasodilators

ACE Inhibitors

Renin, produced by the kidney, converts Angiotensinogen to Angiotensin I, which is converted in the lungs by Angiotensin Converting Enzyme (ACE) to Angiotensin II. Angiotensin II stimulates the adrenal cortex to produce Aldosterone which induces peripheral vasoconstriction. Aldosterone activates the pump in the distal renal tubule leading to reabsorption of sodium and water from urine, in exchange for potassium and hydrogen ions.

ACE Inhibitors may induce cough, angioedema and lichenoid reactions, there may be taste loss with Enalapril and Captopril. Erythema Multiforme may also be induced. Burning mouth has also been reported. NSAIDs should be avoided as the risk of renal damage is increased.

Other vasodilators decrease the blood pressure in hypertension. This decreases the work of the heart in cardiac failure. They may dilate predominantly veins, eg nitrates, or arteries eg hydralazine, or a mixture eg prazosin.

Calcium channel-blockers

These cause coronary and peripheral vessel vasodilation and are negatively inotropic ie they reduce the strength of cardiac contraction. They are antiarrhythmic. Calcium antagonists are used in coronary heart disease and hypertension. Examples include nifedipine and diltiazem.

Oral side-effects include gingival hyperplasia.[9] Headache and flushing may occur, as can peripheral oedema.

Potassium-channel activators

Nicorandil has vasodilating properties on both the arterial and venous sides of the circulation. This drug can produce large ulcers in the mouth[14] that are similar to major aphthae and may be confused with malignancy.

Warfarin

This may be used in the management of atrial fibrillation (as thromboembolic prophylaxis), deep vein thrombosis (DVT), prevention of embolisation secondary to MI and after prosthetic heart valve replacement.

The therapeutic efficacy is monitored using the International Normalised Ratio (INR). There are local variations in what is considered to be a 'safe' INR to carry out surgical dental treatment. This aspect is discussed fully in the chapter relating to bleeding disorders (chapter 9).

The INR should be checked on the day of the procedure. Whenever warfarin dosage is adjusted, the normal regimen is to stop the drug two days before the procedure, with an INR check pre-operatively and resumption

Table 6 American Society of Anaesthesiologists (ASA) Classification
ASA I   Healthy
ASA II   Mild systemic disease - No functional limitation
ASA III Severe systemic disease - Definite functional limitation
ASA IV Severe disease - Constant threat to life
ASA V   Moribund
ASA VI Brain dead patient whose organs are to be removed for donor purposes

Table 7 Prognosis after MI with general anaesthesia

Time Since infarction	Incidence of further infarction after surgery (%)
0-6 months	55
1-2 years	22
2-3 years	6
> 3 years	1
No Infarction	0.66

of the warfarin on the evening of the day of procedure. Adjustment must be in consultation with the patient's physician, and is usually not required.

Heparin

This is an anticoagulant usually used in the hospital setting. It is monitored by the Activated Partial Thromboplastin Time (APTT).

Since the advent of the low molecular weight heparins, some cases of DVT are now treated on a community basis and a dental surgeon in practice could encounter a patient on this form of treatment. Tinzaparin and enoxaparin are two of the more commonly used agents; they have little effect on dental treatment.

GENERAL AND LOCAL ANAESTHESIA, SEDATION AND MANAGEMENT CONSIDERATIONS IN THE DENTAL PATIENT WITH CARDIOVASCULAR DISEASE

The association of oral health and coronary heart disease is controversial. Some studies suggest an association between periodontitis and risk of heart disease.[15] So excellent dental care may play a role in the prevention of cardiovascular conditions.

As alluded to earlier, the key to assessment is the degree of compensation or control of the underlying

disorder that has been achieved. The relevance with regard to anaesthesia of some disorders is discussed earlier. The American Society of Anaesthesiologists (ASA) has developed a system known as the ASA Classification, which is a universally recognised stratification of patient fitness (encompassing all systems of the body). The Classification is shown in *Table 6*.

In hypertensive patients, if feasible, treatment is best carried out under local analgesia, with or without sedation. As mentioned previously both beta-blocking and non-potassium sparing diuretic drugs can exacerbate unwanted effects of epinephrine in dental local anaesthetics and dose reduction of epinephrine is wise. Similarly, patients who have had cardiac transplants may super-react to the cardiac effects of epinephrine in dental local anaesthetics. The use of sedation may be valuable in patients with cardiac disease. Firstly, sedation may reduce the effects of stress. Secondly, the use of sedation may eliminate the need for general anaesthesia. Antihypertensive drugs are not usually stopped before a general anaesthetic.

In patients post myocardial infarction, elective surgery under GA or LA should be postponed for at least

3 months and, ideally, a year. Within 3 months of an MI, even emergency treatment is best carried out with medical consultation. The prognosis after an MI of patients undergoing a GA is shown in *Table 7*.

Aspects relating to the management of patients with cardiovascular disease other than operative pain control measures, include the treatment of conditions secondary to drug therapy and post-operative pain control. Drug problems which may arise include dry mouth which will necessitate a preventive regimen and when severe may require the use of artificial saliva. Drug-induced gingival overgrowth can occur as mentioned earlier as a result of post-transplantation drugs and calcium-channel blockers (Fig. 3). Repeated gingival surgery is not uncommon in such patients.

Normally, post-operative pain in dentistry is controlled by non-steroidal analgesics. However, the use of non-steroidal anti-inflammatory drugs such as aspirin should be avoided in patients taking warfarin as the anti-coagulant effect is increased. Similarly, non-steroidal drugs inhibit the hypotensive effects of anti-hypertensive medication and their nephro-toxicity is increased in the presence of diuretics.

Smoking is a common cause of peri-operative morbidity in the context of GA. In addition to its deleterious respiratory effects, the carbon monoxide produced by cigarettes has a negatively inotropic effect. Nicotine increases the heart rate and systemic arterial blood pressure.

Carbon monoxide decreases oxygen supply and nicotine increases oxygen demand. This is particularly significant in patients with ischaemic heart disease. These patients can get real benefit by stopping smoking 12-24 hours before surgery. The negative respiratory effects of smoking take at least 6 weeks to start to abate.

SUMMARY

There are many factors which need to be borne in mind from the cardio-vascular point of view when assessing the status of a patient requiring dental treatment. The degree of control of the disease, sequelae arising from it and time from the causative event can all be of importance in treatment planning. Much of the information required to make safe decisions will be obtained through a thorough history.

1. Hemsley S M. Drug therapy in dental practice. *Br Dent J* 1984; **157**: 368.
2. Punnia Moorthy A, Coghlan K, O'Neil R. Drug therapy among dental out-patients. *Br Dent J* 1984; **156**: 261.
3. Carter LM, Godlington F L, Meechan J G. Screening for hypertension in dentistry. *J Dent Res* 1997;**76**:1037 Abstract 152.
4. Perusse R, Goulet J-P, Turcotte J-Y. Contra-indications to the use of vasoconstrictors in dentistry. Part I. *Oral Surg* 1992;**74**:679-686.
5. Seymour R A, Lowry R, Whitworth J M, Martin M V. Infective endocarditis, dentistry and antibiotic prophylaxis; time for a rethink? *Br Dent J* 2000;**189**:610-616.
6. NICE Guidelines: Prophylaxis against infective endocarditis. Clinical Guidelines CG64 March 2008.
7. Dessler F A, Roberts W C. Mode of death and type of cardiac disease in opiate addicts: analysis of 168 necroscopy cases. *Am J Cardiol* 1989;**64**:909-920.
8. Ryder W. The electrocardiogram in dental anaesthesia. *Anaesthesia* 1970;**25**:46-62.
9. Thomason J M, Seymour R A, Ellis J S, Kelly P J, Parry G, Dark J. Iatrogenic gingival overgrowth in cardiac transplantation. *J Periodontol* 1995;**66**:742-746.
10. Meechan J G, Parry G, Rattray D T, Thomason J M. Effects of dental local anaesthesia in cardiac transplant recipients. *Br Dent J* 2002;**192**:161-163.
11. Gilbert E M, Eiswirht C C, Mealey P C, Larrabee B S, Herrick C M, Bristow M R. ß-adren-ergic supersensitivity of the transplanted heart is pre-synaptic in origin. *Circulation* 1989;**79**:344-349.
12. Sugimura M, Hirota Y, Shibutani T, Xiwa H, Hori T, Kim Y, Matsuura H. An echocardiographic study of interactions between Pindolol and epinephrine contained in a local anesthetic solution. *Anesthesia Progress* 1995;**42**:29-35.
13. Meechan J G. Plasma potassium changes in hypertensive patients undergoing oral surgery with local anaesthetics containing epinephrine. *Anesthesia Progress* 1997;**44**:106-109.
14. Scully C, Azul A M, Crighton A, Felix D, Field A, Porter S R. Nicorandil can induce severe oral ulceration. *Oral Surg Oral Med Pathol Oral Radiol Endod* 2001; **91**:189-93.
15. Dietrich T, Jimenez M, Krall Kaye E A, Vokonas P S, Garcia R A. Age-dependent associations between chronic periodontitis/edentulism and risk of coronary heart disease. *Circulation* 2008; **117**: 1668-74.

Chapter 2
The respiratory system

M. Greenwood and J. G. Meechan

IN BRIEF

- Respiratory disorders may present with cough, sputum, wheeze or haemoptysis. Differentiation from cardiac disease (which may be concurrent) can be difficult since certain features are common to both. These include dyspnoea, finger clubbing and cyanosis. A thorough history helps in differentiation.
- Respiratory failure can be precipitated in a patient with respiratory impairment if they have a GA. The impairment may be temporary eg due to infection. An upper respiratory tract infection may progress to the chest and therefore a GA should be postponed in the non-urgent case.
- Enquiry should be made regarding the efficacy of medication eg inhalers used in the management of asthma and should be available for use if required. The possibility that the patient may be taking (or have taken) steroids should be borne in mind.
- Patients who are short of breath feel more comfortable in a sitting position rather than supine.

Respiratory disorders are common and their main significance in dentistry relates to intravenous sedation, general anaesthesia and the unwanted effects of prescribed drugs. The degree of compliance achievable for local analgesia may also be compromised. As with most disorders the history is important in the assessment of such patients.

The respiratory system is always affected to some extent by smoking and enquiry should always be made with regard to smoking habits. **Cough** is a non-specific reaction to irritation anywhere from the pharynx to the lungs. It may produce sputum or be non-productive. Haemoptysis (coughing up of blood) may occur and it is important to differentiate this from haematemesis (vomiting of blood). Large volumes of blood may be coughed up in lung cancer, bronchiectasis and tuberculosis. Lesser amounts may be observed in pneumonia and pulmonary embolism. A summary of specific points to obtain in the history is given in *Table 1* and these are discussed further below.

Infections of the respiratory tract may be acute or chronic and may be of the upper (ie vocal cords or above) or lower tract. Infections of either are a contra-indication to GA, which should be deferred until resolution has occurred. An upper respiratory tract infection (URTI) will readily progress to the lower tract if a GA is given. URTIs may occur as part of the common cold, as pharyngitis or tonsillitis and as a laryngotracheitis. The latter in children may cause stridor ('croup').

The **paranasal air sinuses** may become infected secondary to a viral URTI (a viral cause being most common). In acute sinusitis, the most commonly implicated bacteria are *Streptococcus pneumoniae* and *Haemophilus influenzae*. In maxillary sinusitis (which may also occur secondary to periapical infection of intimately related teeth) pain in the cheek and/or upper teeth is worsened by lowering the head and there is a mucopurulent nasal discharge. The maxilla over the antrum is tender to palpation. An occipito-mental radiograph may show increased radiopacity of the antrum but this can often be difficult to assess objectively and may be due to a thickened mucosal lining rather than acute infection (*Fig. 1*). Analgesics and antibiotics eg

Table 1 Points in history of patients with respiratory disease

- Smoking
- Cough
- Sputum (colour)
- Acute problem or chronic disorder?
- Infection - URTI/LRTI
- Sinusitis
- Pneumonia - primary, secondary, atypical
- Asthma
- COPD
- TB
- Bronchiectasis
- Cystic Fibrosis
- Haemoptysis
- Lung Cancer

(Occupational lung disorders, Sarcoidosis, ARDS - may be guided by facts obtained in the earlier history)

GENERAL MEDICINE AND SURGERY FOR DENTAL PRACTITIONERS

amoxicillin, erythromycin or doxycycline for 2 weeks may be required. In chronic sinusitis, formal drainage of the antrum may be required.

Lower respiratory tract infections are often viral, but bacterial infection will frequently supervene. There are signs of systemic upset eg fever, pleuritic pain (sharp pain on inspiration), cough, green/yellow sputum and possibly haemoptysis. The patient (especially the elderly) may appear confused and indeed this may be the only sign that something is wrong. There will often be dyspnoea (the subjective feeling of a shortage of breath).

Primary pneumonia occurs in previously healthy individuals and is often due to pneumococci or 'atypical' organisms. Secondary pneumonias

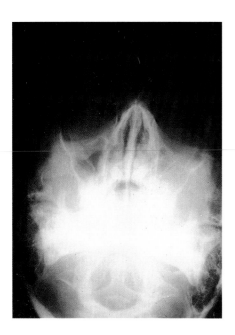

Fig. 1 Increased radiopacity of the left maxillary antrum in maxillary sinusitis

occur in patients with impaired defences eg in malignancy or Chronic Obstructive Pulmonary Disease (COPD) such as chronic bronchitis and emphysema. Atypical pneumonias include *Legionella pneumophila* and *Pneumocystis carinii (jiroveci)* (a protozoan-like cyst) in AIDS. The former organism causes Legionnaire's Disease and the organism multiplies in stagnant water found in air conditioning systems. It has been isolated from dental units which have been unused over a prolonged period eg weekends or holidays.[1] Units such as this should be 'run through' thoroughly before resuming clinical use.

An inadequately treated pneumonia may lead to a lung abscess. Aspiration of a foreign body from the mouth can also be a cause. In dentistry this may occur when a rubber dam is not used when it is indicated leading to inhalation of debris or if an inadequate throat pack or uncuffed endotracheal tube is used for dental procedures under GA. The commonest infecting organisms are *Staphylococcus aureus* or *Klebsiella pneumoniae*.

Bronchial asthma is a generalised airways obstruction which in the early stages is paroxysmal and reversible. The obstruction, leading to wheezing, is due to bronchial muscle contraction, mucosal swelling and increased mucus production. Exposure to allergens and/or stress can induce an attack. It is now accepted that inflammation is an important aetiological factor in asthma and this has resulted in the use of anti-inflammatory medication in the management of the condition.[2] In terms of management, infrequent attacks can be managed by salbutamol (ventolin) inhalers as needed or prophylactically if an attack might be predicted eg before exercise or prior to a stressful event such as dental treatment. If the attacks are more frequent, the salbutamol should be used regularly. If this is insufficient, inhaled steroids (or cromoglycate in the young) should be used. In severe cases systemic steroids may be prescribed. Enquiry should be directed toward the efficacy of medication, use of steroids and whether there have been episodes of hospitalisation.

COPD comprises chronic bronchitis and emphysema. Chronic bronchitis is said to exist when there is sputum production on most days for 3 months of the year in two successive years. Emphysema is dilatation of airspaces distal to the terminal bronchioles by destruction of their walls. The two co-exist in varying proportions in COPD and smoking is a common predisposing factor.[3] Emphysema may rarely be inherited and is then due to Alpha-1-antitrypsin deficiency. Some COPD patients are breathless but not cyanosed ('pink puffers') some are cyanotic and if heart failure supervenes become oedematous or bloated ('blue bloaters'). In these patients the respiratory centres are relatively insensitive to carbon dioxide and they rely on 'hypoxic drive' to maintain respiratory effort. It is dangerous to give high levels of supplemental oxygen for longer than brief periods to these patients as breathing may stop or the patient may begin to hypoventilate.

Treatment of acute exacerbations of COPD involve broad spectrum antibiotics, bronchodilators (inhaled or nebulised) and possibly physiotherapy. Steroids may also be used. Dental treatment should be avoided during an exacerbation and in any event if

Table 2	Extra-pulmonary manifestations of sarcoidosis
General	- fever, malaise, lymphadenopathy, hepatosplenomegaly
Oral	- salivary gland swelling, gingival swelling
Skin	- erythema nodosum
Eye	- enlarged lacrimal glands
Bones	- arthralgia
Heart	- cardiomyopathy
CNS	- cranial and peripheral nerve palsies (especially facial nerve)
Kidney	- renal stones

possible should be carried out under LA.

Tuberculosis caused mainly by *Mycobacterium tuberculosis* is a disease that has increased in prevalence in recent years, largely due to the immunocompromised HIV population, in the malnourished eg the materially deprived and in immigrants from underdeveloped countries. It is unlikely to be a great risk to dental staff unless the patient has an active pulmonary type in which case dental treatment is better deferred until control has been achieved. Pulmonary TB is usually spread by inhaling infected sputum and is highly infectious when active. If delayed treatment is not possible aerosols should be reduced to a minimum and it may be useful to carry out treatment under rubber dam. Masks and spectacles are mandatory for all personnel. Most primary infections are subclinical. Haematogenous spread can lead to skeletal or genitourinary lesions. Widespread lesions give rise to the term 'Miliary TB'. A diagnosis of TB is suggested by chronic cough, haemoptysis, fever, night sweats and weight loss. Confirmatory tests include chest X-ray, sputum examination for acid and alcohol fast bacilli and the skin test or Mantoux test which shows a delayed hypersensitivity to a protein derived from *Mycobacterium tuberculosis*. Specific chemotherapy is by far the most important measure in the treatment of TB. In the UK, rifampicin, isoniazid, ethambutol, streptomycin and pyrazinamide are considered in the first-line treatment of TB. The majority of patients are treated as outpatients whereas a policy of 'isolation' was followed in the past. Immobilisation of the patient is necessary in some forms of skeletal TB.

Bronchiectasis is a condition where the bronchi are irreversibly dilated and act as stagnation areas for persistently infected mucus. It should be suspected in any persistent or recurrent chest infection. It may be congenital eg in cystic fibrosis or post infection eg TB, measles. Haemoptysis may occur. Intensive physiotherapy, antibiotics and bronchodilators are the mainstays of treatment.

Cystic fibrosis is one of the commonest inherited diseases (1 in 2000 live births) and is autosomal recessive. The cells are relatively impermeable to chloride (hence diagnosis by measuring the chloride concentration of sweat) and thus salt-rich secretions are produced. The mucus is viscid and blocks glands. In the young adult or child recurrent chest infections are seen, bronchiectasis and pancreatic insufficiency also occur.

Lung cancer is usually linked to cigarette smoking and may present in various ways including cough and haemoptysis. The disease may produce cerebral and hepatic metastases. The latter produce hepatomegaly, jaundice or ascites (fluid in the abdomen producing distension). Bone metastases (including the facial bones) may lead to pathological fracture. If the superior vena cava becomes compressed by tumour, facial oedema and cyanosis may occur (the Superior Vena Cava Syndrome). These patients may have muscle weakness (the Eaton-Lambert Syndrome) in which, unlike myasthenia gravis the use of muscles leads to better function rather than a deterioration. Ectopic hormone production may occur in lung cancer (commonly adrenocorticotrophic hormone - ACTH).

Occupational lung disease is still seen in patients and may lead to significant respiratory impairment. Most inhaled particles cause no damage as they become trapped in the nose or are removed by the muco-ciliary

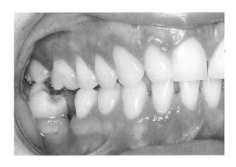

Fig. 2 This young female patient presented with gingivitis but had good oral hygiene. The gingival swelling was later found to be due to sarcoid

clearance system. Particles may be destroyed by alveolar macrophages. The pneumoconioses are conditions which result from inhalation of various dusts and include asbestosis, silicosis and coal workers' pneumoconiosis. They will all restrict respiratory efficiency to some degree and potentially have a bearing on dental treatment provision.

Sarcoidosis is a multi-system disorder of unknown aetiology and is characterised by non-caseating granulomata. It most commonly affects the lungs of young adults but may occur at any age. Thoracic sarcoidosis classically presents incidentally as bilateral hilar lymphadenopathy on chest X-ray and is often asymptomatic. It may, however, be associated with cough, fever, arthralgia, malaise or erythema nodosum. Erythema nodosum comprises painful, erythematous nodular lesions on the anterior shins, but are not specific for sarcoid, for example they may also be seen in TB. Extra-thoracic manifestations of sarcoidosis are listed in *Table 2*. Gingival swelling found to be due to sarcoid is shown in *Fig. 2*. The mainstay of diagnosis is a rise in Serum Angiotensin Converting Enzyme level. Treatment may be carried out using steroids which may have implications for dental treatment as well as potential respiratory impairment.

The **Adult Respiratory Distress Syndrome (ARDS)** is a progressive respiratory insufficiency which usually follows a major systemic insult eg trauma, infection, and is largely due to interstitial pulmonary oedema

arising from leaking capillaries. It is only relevant to mainstream dental practice in that about one third of surviving patients may be left with pulmonary fibrosis. Other causes of pulmonary fibrosis include connective tissue disorders eg rheumatoid arthritis, Sjögren's Syndrome or may be unknown - cryptogenic. Management is difficult and largely relies on immunosuppression eg with prednisolone.

EXAMINATION

The patient's colour may give an early clue as to their condition eg the pink puffer or blue bloated patient with COPD. The patient may be centrally cyanosed with a bluish hue to the tongue/lips. This is seen when there is a deoxygenated haemoglobin level of concentration greater than 5 grams per decilitre. Respiratory disease may cause the patient to be short of breath or tachypnoeic (breathing quickly) at rest or on minimal exertion eg walking into the surgery. The patient may be using their accessory muscles of respiration. In patients who retain carbon dioxide, the radial pulse at the wrist may feel very full and 'bounding' and carbon dioxide retainers may also have a flapping tremor of the hands when they are held outstretched.

Intra-oral examination may reveal that patients using corticosteroid inhalers are predisposed to developing oral/pharyngeal candidosis (*Fig. 3*) and patients using beta$_2$ agonists and antimuscarinic agents often will have a dry mouth. More uncommon

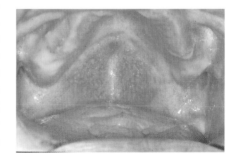

Fig. 3 This patient was using inhaled corticosteroids for the treatment of COPD and has developed candidosis as a result. The full upper denture baseplate has protected the palate more anteriorly

Table 3 Relevant factors on examination of a dental patient with respiratory disease which may be present.

- Colour
- Central cyanosis
- Dyspnoea, tachypnoea, (use of accessory muscles)
- Finger clubbing
- Cervical lymphadenopathy (URTI, TB)
- Bounding pulse
- Oral hyperpigmentation
- Flapping tremor

oral findings on examination may be a hyperpigmentation of the soft palate in lung cancer, or even bony metastases from lung cancer in the jaws. Chronic ulcers of the dorsum of tongue may rarely be an oral manifestation of TB. Cervical lymphadenopathy from TB may also be evident, but the more common lymphadenopathy secondary to a URTI should be considered first, (*Table 3*).

The pulse oximeter gives a guide to the efficiency of oxygenation of blood (*Fig. 4*). It measures the pulse rate and oxygen saturation. The sensor, placed usually on a fingertip contains two Light Emitting Diodes (LEDs), one red measuring the amount of oxygenated haemoglobin, the other infrared, measuring the total haemoglobin. The oxygen saturation is the amount of oxygen carried in the blood relative to the maximum possible amount. There is a linear relationship between oxygen in the blood and the arterial oxygen saturation. Pulse oximetry does not necessarily indicate normal ventilation, since the saturation can appear normal if supplemental oxygen is being used.

RELEVANCE OF DRUGS IN RESPIRATORY DISORDERS

Corticosteroids

The use of corticosteroids, normally by inhalation, can lead to some problems related to dental management. Firstly, the use of steroid inhalers can lead to localised lowered resistance to opportunistic infections. As a

result of this oro-pharyngeal candidal infection may occur.[4] In order to avoid this complication patients should be advised to rinse and gargle with water after use of their inhaler. Secondly, regular use of inhaled steroids can lead to adrenal suppression thus the patient may be at risk of an adrenal crisis if they are subjected to stress.

Beta adrenergic agonist bronchodilators

Beta$_2$ adrenergic agonists such as salbutamol and terbutaline can produce dry mouth, taste alteration and discolouration of the teeth. Dry mouth may increase caries incidence and thus a preventive regimen is important. If the dry mouth is severe artificial saliva may be indicated. The hypokalaemia which may result from large doses of beta$_2$ adrenergic agonists may be exacerbated by a reduction in potassium produced by high doses of steroids and by epinephrine in dental local anaesthetics.

Antimuscarinic bronchodilators

Drugs such as ipratropium can produce dry mouth and taste disturbance and may also cause stomatitis. The absorption of the antifungal agent ketoconazole is decreased during combined therapy with ipratropium.

There is an increased chance of arryhthmia with halogenated general anaesthetic agents during combined therapy with theophylline. In addition theophylline decreases the sedative and anxiolytic effects of some benzodiazepines including diazepam. Plasma theophylline levels are reduced by carbamazepine and phenytoin[5] and increased by erythromycin.[6,7] Theophylline levels may also be affected by corticosteroids. Hydrocortisone and methylprednisolone have been shown to both increase and decrease theophylline levels. Terfenadine decreases the plasma concentration of erythromycin[8] and this may be clinically important.

Anti-muscarinic effects (such as dry mouth) are increased with concurrent use of tricyclic and mono-amine oxidase inhibitor antidepressant drugs.

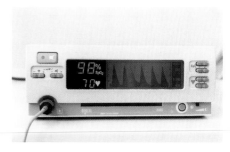

Fig. 4 A standard pulse oximeter

Cromoglycate

Dry mouth, burning mouth and taste disturbance may occur during cromoglycate therapy.

Antihistamines

The more modern antihistamines such as terfenadine may produce dry mouth, but this is less common compared to older antihistamines. Stevens-Johnson syndrome may occur. Tricyclic and mono-amine oxidase inhibitor antidepressants increase anti-muscarinic effects such as dry mouth when used concurrently.

Among the many drugs which may produce dangerous arrythmias when combined with terfenadine are erythromycin,[8] the anti fungal drugs, miconazole, fluconazole, itraconazole and ketoconazole[9] and the antiviral agents efavirenz, indinavir, nelfinavir, ritonavir and saquinavir. Grapefruit juice must be avoided during therapy with terfenadine to avoid arrhythmias.

The antihistamines have an enhanced sedative effect when combined with anxiolytic and hypnotic drugs.

Cough suppressants and decongestants

Occasionally cough suppressants such as codeine may be used by patients and the additive effect of this should be considered when prescribing opioid analgesics (such as paracetamol/codeine compound drugs). There is a theoretical possibility that the adrenergic effects of epinephrine in dental local anaesthetics will be enhanced by ephedrine so dose reduction should be considered. Ephedrine may increase the chance of arrhythmia with halogenated general anaesthetic agents.

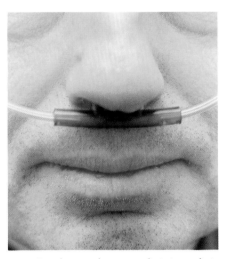

Fig. 5 Supplemental oxygen administered via nasal cannula

RELEVANCE OF RESPIRATORY DISORDERS IN THE PROVISION OF LOCAL ANAESTHESIA, SEDATION, GENERAL ANAESTHESIA AND MANAGEMENT IN DENTAL PRACTICE

Excellent dental care is important in patients with respiratory disorders. There is some evidence of an association of poor dental health with pneumonia and COPD. In addition there is good evidence that improvements in oral hygiene can reduce the impact of respiratory disease in high-risk individuals.[10]

The relevant drug interactions and adverse effects of medication used to treat respiratory disorders have been discussed above. Other effects of respiratory disease on management are considered here. In the presence of respiratory impairment, general anaesthesia can be potentially dangerous since respiratory failure may be precipitated. If infection is temporary then resolution should be awaited. If GA is unavoidable and the condition is chronic eg in cases of COPD or bronchiectasis, then the condition of the patient should be optimised eg using preoperative physiotherapy, sometimes antibiotics, bronchodilators such as salbutamol and antimuscarinics such as Ipratropium (sometimes nebulised). Even when treated using LA, these patients may become dyspnoeic, especially when supine. As part of any preoperative work up, benefit can be gained by stopping smoking.

The use of rubber dam may be unacceptable in patients with COPD due to further compromise of the airway. If rubber dam is necessary supplemental oxygen via a nasal cannula may be required but low concentrations should be used. *Fig. 5* shows a patient receiving supplemental oxygen via a nasal cannula.

In cases of active TB, a GA is contra-indicated, both due to impaired respiratory function or contamination of anaesthetic machine circuits. Asthmatic patients should have treatment carried out using LA if possible. Effort should be made to allay anxiety as far as possible and treatment should not be carried out if the patient has not brought their normal medication and such medication is otherwise unavailable. Relative analgesia using nitrous oxide and oxygen is preferred to intravenous sedation since the former can be rapidly controlled. GA can be complicated by hypoxia and increased carbon dioxide which can lead to pulmonary oedema even if cardiac function is normal.

As mentioned above patients may not be comfortable in the supine position if they have respiratory problems.

If the patient suffers from asthma then aspirin-like compounds should not be prescribed as many asthmatic patients are allergic to these analgesics.[11] A severe asthmatic attack can be life-threatening and as stress may contribute to the onset of such a condition the dentist should have the equipment to deal with such an emergency at hand. A salbutamol inhaler or nebulised salbutamol are useful.

Intravenous hydrocortisone and intravenous aminophylline are reserved for patients who do not respond quickly to nebulised bronchodilator therapy. Care is needed with patients already taking theophymlline preparations and this step is best left until medical assistance is available.

The use of **supplemental steroids** prior to dental surgery in patients at risk of an 'adrenal crisis' is a contentious issue. The rationale for steroid supplementation is as follows.

Corticosteroids are critical in the body's response to trauma (including operative trauma). A normal response is to increase corticosteroid production in response to stress. If this response is absent, hypotension, collapse and death will occur. The hypothalamo-pituitary-adrenal axis will fail to function if either pituitary or adrenal cortex ceases to function eg administration of corticosteroids leads to negative feedback to the hypothalamus causing decreased ACTH production and adrenocortical atrophy. This atrophy means that an endogenous steroid boost cannot be produced in response to stress. Recent studies have suggested that dental surgery may not require supplementation.[12] More invasive procedures however, such as third molar surgery or the treatment of very apprehensive patients may still require cover. It is wise, even if supplementary steroids have not been used, to monitor the blood pressure of patients taking steroids. If the diastolic pressure falls by more than 25% then a steroid injection (100 mg hydrocortisone) is indicated. Patients who may require supplementation are those who are currently taking corticosteroids or have done so in the last month. A supplement may also be required if steroid therapy has been used for more than one month in the previous year. If the patient is receiving the equivalent of 20 mg prednisolone daily then extra supplementation is not required.

SUMMARY

Respiratory problems affect many aspects of dental treatment. Eliciting a proper history from the patient with respiratory disease will help prevent serious problems and alert the dentist to oro-facial conditions which may result from the use of appropriate medication. Patients with significant respiratory problems, particularly if they need extensive treatment are best treated in the hospital setting.

1. Scully C, Cawson R A, Griffiths M. Occupational hazards to dental staff. *BDJ* publication 1990; 178-179.

2. Randall T. International consensus report urges sweeping reform in asthma treatment. *JAMA* 1992; **267:** 2153-2154.

3. Lee P N, Fry J S, Forey B A. Trends in lung cancer, chronic obstructive lung disease, and emphysema death rates for England and Wales 1941-1985 and their relation to trends in cigarette smoking. *Thorax* 1990; **45:** 657-665.

4. McAllen M K, Kochanowski S J, Shaw K M. Steroid aerosols in asthma: an assessment of betamethasone valerate and a 12-month study of patients on maintenance treatment. *Br Med J* 1974; i:171.

5. Reed R C, Schwartz H J. Phenytoin-theophylline-quinidine interaction. *New Engl J Med* 1983; 308 724-725.

6. Reisz G, Pingleton S K, Melethil S, Ryan P. The effect of erythromycin on theophylline pharmacokinetics in chronic bronchitis. *Am Rev Resp Dis* 1983; **127:** 581-584.

7. Paulsen O, Hoglund P, Nilsson L-G, Bengtsson H-I. The interaction of erythromycin with theophylline. *Eur J Clin Pharmacol* 1987; **32:** 493-498.

8. Honig P K, Woosley R L, Zamani K, Conner D P, Cantilena L R. Changes in the pharmacokinetics and electrocardiographic pharmacodynamics of terfenadine with concomitant adminstration of erythromycin. *Clin Pharmacol Ther* 1992; **52:** 231-238.

9. Eller M G and Okerholm R A. Pharmacokinetic interaction between terfenadine and keto-conazole. *Clin Pharmacol Ther* 1991; **49:** 130.

10. Azarpazhooh A, Leake J L. Systematic review of the association between respiratory diseases and oral health. *J Periodontol* 2006; **77:** 1465-482

11. Szczeklik A. The cyclo-oxygenase theory of aspirin-induced asthma. *Eur Resp J* 1990; **3:** 588-593.

12. Thomason J M, Girdler N M, Kendall-Taylor P, Wastell H, Weddell, A. Seymour R A. An investigation into the need for supplementary steroids in organ transplant patients undergoing gingival surgery. *J Clin Period* 1992; **26:** 577-582.

Chapter 3
The gastrointestinal system

M. Greenwood and J. G. Meechan

IN BRIEF

- Cervical lymph node enlargement is most commonly caused by infection. Neoplasms (local or systemic) may also be responsible.
- Peptic ulceration (related to infection with *Helicobacter pylori*) is a contra-indication to non-steroidal anti-inflammatory drugs. Care is also needed with steroid therapy which can lead to peptic ulcer bleeding.
- Anaemia may occur secondary to blood loss from a gastrointestinal cause.
- Vomiting after GA may occur in some gastric disorders leading to an inhalation pneumonitis. Gastric reflux may produce dental erosion.
- Dysphagia (difficulty swallowing) is a symptom which should always be taken seriously.

Diseases of the gastrointestinal (GI) system can be relevant to the dental surgeon for several reasons. The mouth may display signs of the disease itself, for example the cobblestone mucosa, facial or labial swelling of Crohn's disease, or the osteomata of Gardner's syndrome. These are well covered elsewhere and not discussed further here. The sequelae of GI disease, for example gastric reflux producing dental erosion, iron deficiency anaemia and treatment such as corticosteroid therapy may all have a bearing on management and choice of anaesthesia.

RELEVANT POINTS IN HISTORY

Lethargy, dyspnoea and angina may all occur secondary to **anaemia** from a gastro-intestinal cause, but cardio-respiratory causes should also be borne in mind. The cause of an anaemia should always be investigated. The possibility of blood loss from the GI tract should be considered. Weight loss may be due to reduced nutritional intake secondary to anorexia, nausea or vomiting. There may be loss of protein from diseased bowel eg in ulcerative colitis. Cancer of the GI tract is the most significant potential cause of weight loss. The quantity and time course of the weight loss are both important. Enquiry with regard to appetite and any changes should also be made.

'**Heartburn** or '**indigestion**' are vague terms often used by patients and may be used to describe upper abdominal pain, gastro-oesophageal regurgitation, anorexia, nausea and vomiting. **Oesophageal reflux** or 'heartburn' causes epigastric pain ie abdominal pain around the lower end of the sternum, which radiates to the back and is worse on stooping and drinking hot drinks. It can have implications for general anaesthesia (see below) and can be a cause of dental erosion[1] especially on the palatal/lingual surfaces of the teeth[2] due to the acidity of the gastric fluid. Factors promoting gastro-oesophageal reflux are shown in *Table 1*.

Dysphagia, or difficulty in swallowing, is a symptom which should always be taken seriously. **Plummer-Vinson** Syndrome is the name given to dysphagia associated with webs of tissue in the pharynx and upper oesophagus. Other components of the syndrome include glossitis, iron deficiency anaemia and koilonychia (spoon-shaped fingernails suggesting iron deficiency but may also occur in

Table 1 Factors promoting Gastro-oseophageal Reflux

- Hiatus hernia
- Pregnancy
- Obesity
- Cigarettes
- Alcohol
- Fatty food

ischaemic heart disease). A patient with koilonychia is shown in *Fig. 1*. Some other causes of dysphagia are listed in *Table 2*.

Vomiting may be due to extra-intestinal causes such as meningitis, migraine or as a result of drug therapy eg morphine. In children, vomiting can be a sign of infection of various body systems. Nausea or vomiting in the morning may be seen in pregnancy, alcoholism and anxiety. Haematemesis, or vomiting of blood, may arise from bleeding oesophageal varices. The relevance to dentistry is mainly related to the fact that these varices may occur secondary to chronic liver disease with its attendant possible implications for blood clotting and drug metabolism due to hepatic impairment.

A current or past history of **peptic ulcer** may be of relevance, particularly when non-steroidal anti-inflammatory drugs (NSAIDs) are being considered. These ulcers are common, affecting around 10% of the world population[3]. Men are affected twice as much as women. The incidence is declining in developed countries; this may be due to dietary changes[4]. Peptic ulcers may affect the lower oesophagus, stomach and duodenum. The pendulum has swung away from surgery for these conditions since the advent of effective drug therapy. *Helicobacter pylori* (a micro-aerophilic Gram negative bacterium) can be identified in

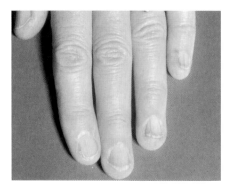

Fig. 1 Koilonychia (spoon-shaped fingernails) in iron deficiency anaemia

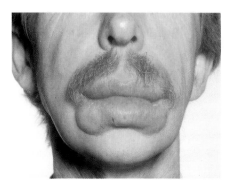

Fig. 2 A patient with Crohn's Disease and consequent marked labial swelling

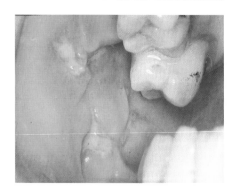

Fig. 3 Recurrent oral ulceration in Crohn's Disease

the gastric antral mucosa in 90% of cases of duodenal ulcers and in the body or antral mucosa of about 60% of cases of gastric ulcer and is a common aetiological factor in peptic ulcer

Table 2 Possible Causes of Dysphagia
Oral causes
Stomatitis Aphthous ulcers Herpetic infection Oral malignancy Xerostomia Tonsillitis Pharyngitis Infections involving fascial spaces of neck
Obstruction in oesophageal wall
Oesophagitis Carcinoma of oesophagus Pharyngeal pouch Oesophageal web - Plummer-Vinson Syndrome (Iron deficiency, post-cricoid web)
External compression of oesophagus
Enlarged neighbouring lymph nodes Left atrial dilatation in mitral stenosis
Disorders of neuromuscular function
Myaesthenia Gravis Muscular dystrophy Stroke Achalasia (failure of oesophageal peristalsis and failure of relaxation of lower oespohageal sphincter)
Other
Foreign body Scleroderma Benign stricture secondary to gastro-oespohageal reflux Globus hystericus (psychogenic)

disease. Triple therapy regimens are used for treatment eg a proton pump inhibitor such as omeprazole, a broad spectrum antibiotic eg amoxycilin and metronidazole when *H.pylori* is involved (see later).

The term **inflammatory bowel disease** includes ulcerative colitis, Crohn's disease (*Figs. 2, 3*) and an indeterminate type. Factors which impact on dental practice include the possibility of anaemia secondary to chronic bleeding and corticosteroid therapy in these patients. Extra-intestinal manifestations of inflammatory bowel disease may occur and are listed in *Table 3*.

A history of GI surgery may give clues to nutritional deficiencies which may be present eg iron, vitamin B_{12} or folate deficiency post gastric surgery. Recurrent oral ulceration and glossitis may ensue.

Pancreatic disease is of relevance in a thorough history since consequent malabsorption of vitamin K may lead to a bleeding tendency. There is also a possibility of diabetes mellitus or a diabetic tendency. Excessive alcohol intake can be a cause of acute pancreatitis and a thorough social history may uncover this information. Other causes of acute pancreatitis include gallstones and some viral infections eg HIV and mumps. Chronic pancreatitis is of a similar aetiology to acute pancreatitis. Endocrine and exocrine function both deteriorate. In both types of pancreatitis, abdominal pain is severe. **Pancreatic cancer** frequently involves the head of the pancreas and local invasion leads to biliary obstruction, diabetes mellitus and pancreatitis. Thrombophlebitis migrans (peripheral vein thrombosis) is a common complication. Pancreactic cancer has the worst prognosis of any cancer in general terms and treatment is usually surgical and palliative.

The patient may give a history of **jaundice** or may actually be jaundiced. Jaundice may be 'pre-hepatic' eg haemolysis, hepatic eg hepatitis (see Chapter 5) or obstructive due to either gallstones or cancer of the head of the pancreas. Patients with

Table 3 Extra-intestinal manifestations of inflammatory bowel disease
Aphthous stomatitis
Hepatic
Fatty change Amyloidosis Gallstones
Skin
Erythema nodosum Pyoderma gangrenosum
Arthritis
Finger clubbing
Eye lesions eg conjunctivitus
Vasculitis
Cardiovascular disease
Broncho-pulmonary disease

obstructive jaundice give a history of generalised itching and passing dark urine and pale stools. The relevance of obstructive jaundice is discussed later.

Congenital disorders of relevance can occur. Familial Polyposis has an incidence of 1 in 24,000 and is transmitted as autosomal dominant. People with the condition have rectal and colonic polyps, and a variant is Gardner's syndrome which also includes bony osteomata and soft tissue tumours eg epidermal cysts. The colonic polyps are premalignant and careful follow up of these patients is needed. Subtotal colectomy with fulguration of rectal polyps may be carried in order to prevent malignancy. Peutz-Jegher's Syndrome is an autosomal dominant condition comprising intestinal polyps and pigmented freckles periorally extending on to the oral mucosa (*Fig. 4*). The gastric and duodenal polyps have a predisposition to become malignant.

Some **skin disorders** may occur as part of a wider picture of GI disease. **Erythema nodosum** and **pyoderma gangrenosum** can occur in inflammatory bowel disease. The skin lesions are painful, erythematous nodular lesions on the anterior shin in erythema nodosum. Bluish edged ulcers occur on the back, thigh and buttocks in pyoderma gangrenosum. The skin disease associated with coeliac disease is dermatitis herpetiformis and comprises an itchy papulovesicular rash mainly on the trunk and upper limbs. IgA deposits at the epithelium basement membrane zone help to establish the diagnosis. There may

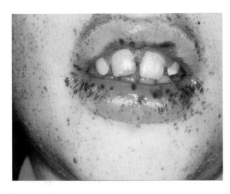

Fig. 4 Peutz-Jegher's Syndrome.

also be papillary tip micro-abscess formation. There may be intra-oral lesions which may be erosive or vesicular and resemble pemphigoid. Treatment is usually with dapsone. Aphthous ulcers may occur.

Coeliac disease is a permanent intolerance to gluten leading to intestinal villous atrophy and GI malabsorption. The villous atrophy reverses when taking a gluten free diet. The disease may be complicated by anaemia and GI lymphoma.

Pseudomembranous colitis can be caused by many antibiotics particularly clindamycin and lincomycin and results from proliferation of toxigenic Clostridium difficile. It is characterised by painful diarrhoea with mucus passage and is treated with oral vancomycin or metronidazole.

A summary of relevant points in the history is given in *Table 4*.

EXAMINATION

Oral lesions as a manifestation of GI disease are well discussed elsewhere and are not considered further here. It is worth remembering that **cervical lymph node enlargement** is an important sign not to be ignored. Possible causes include infection and neoplasia (primary or secondary).

Pallor can be a very subjective way of trying to assess for anaemia. The mucosa at the reflection in the inferior fornix of the eye is the best site for examination. The patient may readily become dyspnoeic secondary to anaemia but this should be considered with an open mind because, as mentioned earlier, cardio-respiratory conditions are more likely to present in this manner.

A patient may be jaundiced for 'extra-hepatic' reasons such as gallstones, cancer of the bile ducts or cancer of the head of pancreas. The sclera is a good site for examining for the yellow tint of jaundice (*Fig. 5*).

Examining the hands may reveal spoon-shaped fingernails or koilonychia (*Fig. 1*). The fingers may be clubbed. Gastro-intestinal causes of clubbing include inflammatory bowel disease (especially Crohn's), cirrhosis, malabsorption and GI lymphoma.

Table 4 Relevant points in the history
General enquiry eg lethargy, anaemia, weight loss, appetite
Dyspepsia, reflux
Dysphagia
Vomiting, haematemesis
Peptic ulcer (current/past)
Inflammatory bowel disease
History of GI surgery
Pancreatic disease
Congenital disorders

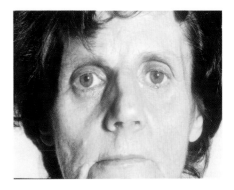

Fig. 5 A jaundiced patient with yellow sclera.

An enlarged lymph node in the left supraclavicular fossa (Virchow's Node, Troisier's Sign) can be a sign of stomach cancer. Anaemia or obstructive jaundice may complicate treatment.

DRUGS USED IN GI DISEASE

Antacids

These are used in ulcer and non-ulcer dyspepsia and in reflux oesophagitis. They are usually aluminium and magnesium containing compounds or alginates. These preparations interfere with the absorption of many drugs including fluoride, ketoconazole, metronidazole and tetracycline.[5] Aluminium hydroxide increases the excretion of aspirin and can reduce the plasma concentration of the analgesic to non-therapeutic levels.[6] It has been shown that maintaining antacids in the mouth for a period before swallowing can counteract reductions in oral pH produced by acidic materials and it has been suggested that this might help counteract the erosion produced by gastro-intestinal reflux.[7]

Drugs altering gut motility eg antispasmodics

These are used in non-ulcer dyspepsia, irritable bowel syndrome and diverticular disease eg hyoscine, mebeverine (anti-muscarinic) tend to decrease motility. Anti-muscarinics produce dry mouth and hyoscine reduces the absorption of the antifungal drug ketoconazole. Drugs such as metoclopramide and domperidone increase motility. The antimuscarinic drug propantheline bromide delays the absorption of paracetamol.[8]

Ulcer healing drugs

Proton pump inhibitors eg omeprazole, lansoprazole

These block the proton pump of the parietal cell. Side effects can include erythema multiforme, stomatitis and dry mouth. Omeprazole increases the anticoagulant effect of warfarin but this is usually unimportant clinically.[10] Omeprazole inhibits the metabolism of diazepam and increases the sedative effect of the latter drug.[11]

Drugs used in inflammatory bowel disease

For the acute condition, topical steroids may be given as enemas. In more extensive situations, oral corticosteroids may be prescribed, leading to intravenous steroids in the most severe cases. Sulphasalazine (a combination of sulphaphyridine and 5-amino salicylic acid) may be given. Similar alternatives include mesalazine and olsalazine. Azathiophrine is used in resistant cases.

Pancreatic supplements

These may be used in cystic fibrosis and chronic pancreatitis. Pancreatin ('Creon') is inactivated by gastric acid and is therefore best taken with food. It can irritate the oral mucosa if held in the mouth. Pancreatin assists in the digestion of starch, fat and protein.

EFFECTS OF GASTROINTESTINAL DISEASE ON LOCAL ANAESTHESIA, SEDATION, GENERAL ANAESTHESIA AND MANAGEMENT IN DENTAL PRACTICE

The principal features of the GI system which may have a bearing on general anaesthesia include obesity, anaemia, reflux/vomiting and the effects of drug therapy.

In the case of obesity, this is not always simply related to diet since physiological and genetic factors are also involved. It is significant in that careful consideration needs to be given to the choice of anaesthesia, and may preclude general anaesthesia on a day case basis. To ensure effective assessment and communication between health care professionals the Body Mass Index (BMI) is used. This is the weight in kilograms divided by the height in metres (squared) ie

$$BMI = \frac{weight}{(height)^2}.$$

Grade 1 is a BMI of 25-30, Grade 2 is 30-40, Grade 3 is more than 40.

After appropriate investigation as to the cause and nature of any anaemia, patients who have developed an iron deficiency anaemia and are awaiting surgery should be treated with oral iron supplements. Blood transfusion would only rarely be indicated in this context. Transfusion less than 48 hours before surgery should be avoided as the oxygen carrying capacity of stored blood is poor.

Certain groups of patients are at risk of aspiration of stomach contents on induction of anaesthesia. These include patients with a history suggestive of hiatus hernia, all non-fasted patients, pregnant patients (stomach emptying is slowed and the cardiac sphincter relaxed). Aspiration is likely to lead to a pneumonitis (Mendelson's Syndrome).

Patients who suffer from reflux of gastro-intestinal contents are at risk of erosion of dental hard tissue. This is particularly the case on the palatal and lingual surfaces. In addition such patients may not be entirely comfortable in the fully supine position and this should be borne in mind during treatment in the dental chair.

Patients with pancreatic disease eg pancreatitis, pancreatic cancer, may have a bleeding tendency due to vitamin K malabsorption (pancreatitis) or biliary obstruction (cancer, especially if there are hepatic metastases). Diabetes mellitus may complicate either pancreatitis or pancreatic cancer as mentioned earlier.

When the patient gives a history suggesting obstructive jaundice, the main risk in safe dental management relates to the risk of excessive bleeding again resulting from vitamin K malabsorption. When possible, surgery should be deferred. If delay is not possible, treatment in hospital with vitamin K supplementation if advised.

Patients with obstructive jaundice are particularly prone to develop renal failure after general anaesthesia (the Hepato-Renal Syndrome). It is thought that this may be due to the toxic effect of bilirubin on the kidney. If at all possible GA should be avoided in these patients. In emergencies (which would be very rare in dentistry) management of these patients depends on maintaining good hydration immediately prior to the GA and using the osmotic diuretic mannitol.

Drug interactions of relevance to dental practice were mentioned above. In addition to drug interactions the prescription of drugs for the treatment of oro-dental conditions may be influenced by the underlying disease.[12] For example the use of non-steroidal anti-inflammatory drugs such as aspirin is contra-indicated in individuals with peptic ulceration. Similarly, the prescription of systemic steroids should be avoided in patients with peptic ulcers as this may lead to perforation leading to pain and blood loss.

The side effects of long-term steroid therapy were discussed in Chapter 2. The longer the patient is on steroid therapy and the higher the dose, the greater the risk of complications. Although steroids are used in GI disease, the duration is usually limited, with maintenance being achieved via other medications.

SUMMARY

As with many other conditions, disorders of the GI tract impact on dentistry. Some conditions lead to dental disease, drugs used in the management of GI disease can produce orofacial signs and symptoms and the prescription of drugs to treat dental conditions is influenced by some underlying disorders.

1. Moazzez R, Barlett D, Anggiansah A. Dental erosion, gastro-oesophageal reflux disease and saliva: how are they related? *J Dent*. 2004; **32:** 489-94.
2. Bartlett D W, Evans D F, Anggiansah A, Smith B G. A study of the association between gastro-oesophageal reflux and palatal dental erosion. *Br Dent J*. 1996; **181:** 125-131.
3. Lam S K. Aetiological factors of peptic ulcer: perspectives of epidemiological observations this century. *J Gastroenterol Hepatol* 1994; **9:** S93-S98.
4. Hollander D, Tarnawaski A. Dietary essential fatty acids and the decline in peptic ulcer disease - a hypothesis. *Gut* 1986; **27:** 239-242.
5. Michel J C, Sayer R J, Kirby W M M Effect of food and antacids on blood levels of Aureomycin and Terramycin. *J Lab Clin Med* 1950; **36:**632
6. Shastri RA. Effect of antacids on salicylate kinetics. *Int J Clin Pharmacol Ther Tox* 1985; **23:** 480-4.
7. Meurman J H, Kuittinen T, Kangas M, Tuisku T. Buffering effects of antacids in the mouth - a new treatment of dental erosion? *Scand J Dent Res* 1988; **96:** 412-417.
8. Nimmo J, Heading R C, Tothill P, Prescott L F. Pharmacological modification of gastric emptying: effects of propantheline and metoclopromide on paracetamol absorption. *Br Med J* 1973; **1:** 587.
9. Noble D W, Smith K J, Dundas C R. Effects of H-2 antagonists on the elimination of bupivacaine. *Br J Anaesth* 1987; **59:** 735-737.
10. Unge P, Svedberg L-E, Nordgren A, Blom H, Andersson T, Lagerstrom P-O, Idstrom J-P. A study of the interaction of omeprazole and warfarin in anticoagulated patients. *Br J Clin Pharmacol* 1992; **34:** 509-512.
11. Gugler R, Jensen J C. Omeprazole inhibits elimination of diazepam. *Lancet* 1984; **i:** 969.
12. British National Formulary. Online at http://bnf.org.

Chapter 4
Neurological disorders

M. Greenwood and J. G. Meechan

IN BRIEF

- Neurological disorders may present in various ways including sensory disturbance, paralysis, altered level of consciousness, fits, speech disturbance, changes in muscle tone or bulk and tremor.
- Facial paralysis may be caused by stroke (upper motor neurone) or Bell's Palsy (lower motor neurone). Surgery in the region of the facial nerve, particularly parotid surgery may also cause dysfunction of the nerve.
- Facial sensory loss (trigeminal nerve) may be caused by extracranial nerve injury. Other causes include multiple sclerosis, stroke and tumours.
- Patients with epilepsy may severely damage the oro-facial tissues in Grand Mal attacks. A good history will alert the practitioner to those who are poorly controlled.
- Some of the drugs used for the treatment of neurological disorders impact on dental disease and its management.
- In patients with severe or complex neurological disorders, consideration should be given to referring such patients for management in a hospital setting.

There are a number of neurological conditions that may be encountered in dental practice. It is important that a dental practitioner has a broad knowledge of the main neurological conditions since they may affect the provision of dental treatment. In addition the first presentation of a neurological disturbance may be a symptom for which the patient seeks a dental opinion. Some malignant disease may present to the dentist as a neurological complaint such as a numb chin.[1]

RELEVANT POINTS IN THE HISTORY

The patient may give a history of 'blackouts'. It is important to be precise about what a patient means by this term as this can indicate anything from a loss of consciousness (LOC) to dizziness. When a history of blackouts is given, information obtained from a witness might be useful. The more that is known about the nature of such an event, the better it can be anticipated and effectively managed (or prevented).

The main points in the history are summarised in *Table 1*.

Syncope may be vaso-vagal in origin (the **simple faint**) or may occur in response to certain situations such as coughing. A vaso-vagal attack may be precipitated by the fear of dental treatment, heat or a lack of food. It occurs due to a reflex bradycardia and peripheral vasodilation. Onset is not instantaneous and the patient will look pale, often feel sick and notice a 'closing in' of visual fields. It cannot occur when a patient is lying down and placing the patient flat with legs raised is the treatment. Jerking of limbs may occur. In carotid sinus syncope, hypersensitivity of the carotid sinus may cause syncope to occur on turning the head. Unlike vaso-vagal syncope this may happen in the supine position.

Patients may suffer from **epilepsy**. If this presents as a blackout the most likely type is Grand Mal. A description of the fit is useful as this may enable early recognition. Precipitating factors should be asked about, as should questioning about altered breathing, cyanosis or tongue biting during a fit. The latter is virtually a diagnostic feature of this type of epilepsy. Medication taken and its efficacy should be assessed in terms of the degree of control achieved. Tonic-clonic or Grand Mal epilepsy is classically preceded by a warning or aura which may comprise an auditory, olfactory or a visual hallucination. A loss of consciousness follows leading to convulsions and subsequent recovery. The patient may be incontinent during a fit. The 'tonic phase' gives way to a 'clonic phase' in which there is repetitive jerky movements, increased salivation and marked bruxism. After a fit of this type, a patient may sleep for up to 12 hours. If the fit continues for more than 5 minutes or continues without a proper end point, 'status epilepticus' is said to be present. This is an emergency situation which requires urgent intervention with a benzodiazepine eg buccal midazolam[2] or intravenous diazepam.

Absence seizures or 'Petit Mal'

Table 1 Main points in the history in the dental patient with possible neurological disorders

- Blackouts, syncope
- Epilepsy
- Stroke, Transient Ischaemic Attack
- Multiple Sclerosis
- Facial pain
- Parkinson's Disease
- Motor Neurone Disease
- Cranial Nerve problems (especially Bell's Palsy)

tend to occur in children who may suddenly arrest speech, attention and movement. So-called 'partial' seizures may be simple or complex. Simple seizures consist of clonic movements of a group of muscles or a limb. Complex seizures may involve hallucinations of hearing, sight or taste.

Febrile convulsions are common in infancy and do not predict progression to later epilepsy. Keeping the child cool with fans, paracetamol and sponging with tepid water are the mainstays of treatment.

Stokes-Adams attacks describe losses of consciousness occurring as a result of cardiac arrhythmias. These may happen with the patient in any position and may occur with no warning except for an awareness of palpitations. Recovery is usually within seconds. Other potential causes of 'blackouts' are shown in *Table 2*.

The patient may give a history of a stroke (**Cerebrovascular Accident - CVA**) or a so-called mini-stroke (**Transient Ischaemic Attack - TIA**). A CVA may be haemorrhagic (subarachnoid, cerebral), thrombotic or embolic in origin. A subarachnoid haemorrhage results from rupture of a Berry aneurysm of the Circle of Willis (which lies at the base of the brain). Subarachnoid haemorrhages tend to affect a younger age group than the other types of CVA and typically patients give a history of a sudden onset of excruciatingly severe headache. The prognosis is poor, but has been improved by surgical and radiological obliteration of the aneurysm. Hypertension and atherosclerosis are contributory factors to other types of CVA. Cerebral thrombosis deprives the brain of part of its blood supply and is the most common type of stroke. Emboli leading to stroke can arise on the wall of an atrium that is fibrillating or from the wall of a heart damaged after a myocardial infarction. Typical results of a CVA are a sudden loss of consciousness, hemiplegia (on the opposite side to the cerebral lesion) and there may be a loss of speech or slurred speech when the CVA affects the left side of

the brain. TIA's comprise a sudden onset of focal CNS signs or symptoms due to a temporary occlusion of part of the cerebral circulation. They are frequently associated with partial or complete stenosis of the carotid artery system. The symptoms resolve in less than 24 hours (usually much more quickly). They are harbingers of a CVA and the known patient will usually be taking prophylactic aspirin.

Patients with **Multiple Sclerosis** have a diverse condition comprising neurological signs and symptoms that are disseminated in both site and time. A viral aetiology has been postulated but the cause is not known. Onset is variable but optic neuritis can lead to visual disturbance or blindness, which may be a presenting feature. Weakness or paralysis of a limb can occur. Nystagmus (jerky, oscillating movement of the eyes - which can also be physiological) may occur, as may ataxia (uncoordinated movements) and dysphagia. Loss of sphincter control leading to urinary incontinence may occur. The diagnosis should be considered in a young patient presenting with trigeminal neuralgia or a facial palsy. Enquiry in such cases should be directed towards other areas to check for neurological signs or symptoms elsewhere.

FACIAL PAIN

Facial pain is common and may affect up to 50% of the elderly population.[3] A paroxysm of excruciating stabbing pain lasting only seconds, in the trigeminal nerve distribution suggests **trigeminal neuralgia**,[4] particularly in patients over 50 years of age. In the vast majority of cases it is unilateral and most commonly affects the mandibular and maxillary divisions. Often a 'trigger area' may be identified from the history that is stimulated by washing or shaving for example. Talking may be enough to stimulate the pain. Usually the trigger is easily identified. Carbamazepine or phenytoin are the mainstays of treatment.

Other neurological causes of facial pain include **post-herpetic neuralgia** and **atypical facial pain**. In post-herpetic neuralgia the patient complains

of a burning pain (often in the ophthalmic division of the trigeminal nerve), which may become chronic. There is no really successful treatment, transcutaneous nerve sectioning and LA infiltration in the painful area has been tried as has carbamazepine. Tricyclic antidepressants have also been used.

When all other causes (including non-neurological causes of facial pain) have been excluded, some patients may still complain of facial pain - usually unilateral. The pain is described as severe, constant and not relieved by analgesics. This type of pain is more common in young females and many are prescribed antidepressants (although not always to curative effect). Atypical facial pain is the term applied to this type of facial pain.

OTHER DISORDERS

Parkinson's Disease results from degeneration of the pigmented cells of the substantia nigra leading to dopamine deficiency. The incidence is equal in males and females. The disease may also result from previous head injury or cerebrovascular disease. Clinically the patient may have tremor in the arms and hands (the latter being described as 'pill-rolling'). A so-called 'cog-wheel' type of rigidity may be seen on movement. Slow movements (bradykinesia) and restlessness (akathisia) may also be noted. The patient may have an expressionless face and a stooped posture. Impaired autonomic function may lead to a postural drop in blood pressure and hypersalivation resulting in drooling of saliva.

Motor Neurone Disease comprises a group of disorders that affect motor neurones at various levels. There is no sensory loss and this helps differentiation from multiple sclerosis. The aetiology is unknown, but a viral agent is thought possible. Oral hygiene may be difficult in these patients and dysphagia and drooling may occur.

Tumours may arise in various components of the CNS and may be primary or metastatic, the latter being more common in the brain. Benign

Table 2 Possible causes of loss of consciousness or 'Blackout'		
Vaso-Vagal Syncope	-	Simple faint
'Situational' Syncope	-	Cough Micturition Carotid sinus hypersensitivity
Epilepsy		
Hypoglycaemia		
Transient Ischaemic Attack		
Orthostatic Hypotension	-	On standing from lying Signifies inadequate vasomotor reflexes eg elderly patients on tablets to lower blood pressure
'Drop attacks'	-	Sudden weakness of legs usually resolved spontaneously
Stokes-Adams Attacks	-	Transient arrhythmia
Anxiety		
Menieres Disease	-	Vertigo, tinnitus, hearing loss
Choking		

brain tumours are still a significant problem as they may cause pressure effects and may not be amenable to surgery due to their site. Headaches are characteristically worse in the morning. Tumours from which cerebral metastases arise include lung, breast, GIT and kidney.

Impairment of vision may occur and this may vary from mild disability to complete blindness. Diplopia or double vision may occur after a 'blowout' fracture of the orbital floor[5] or injury to cranial nerves III, IV and VI. Transient visual disturbance may occur secondary to local anaesthetic that has tracked to the inferior orbital fissure.

Myasthenia Gravis (MG) is an antibody-mediated autoimmune disease with a deficiency of functioning muscle acetylcholine receptors that leads to muscle weakness. The disorder more commonly affects young women. The muscle weakness is progressive and develops rapidly. Some cases are associated with the Eaton-Lambert Syndrome that may occur in some patients with lung or other cancers. In the Eaton-Lambert syndrome, however, the muscles get stronger rather than weaker with activity.

A facial palsy may have a known cause or be idiopathic (*Table 3*). If the cause is not known the name **Bell's Palsy** (*Fig. 1*) is applied. Other causes must be excluded before this term is used. In Bell's Palsy the onset is rapid, unilateral and there may be an ache beneath the ear. The weakness worsens over one to two days. If presentation is early, most clinicians give Prednisolone for 5 days, the aim being to reduce neuronal oedema. An eye patch is of value to protect the cornea. The paralysis is of a lower motor neurone type in which all the facial muscles are affected on that side. In an upper motor neurone lesion eg stroke, the forehead is spared since this region is bilaterally represented in the cortex. Looking for 'forehead sparing' is thus a way of differentiating between upper and lower motor neurone causes of facial weakness.

Bilateral facial paralysis is rare. It may be seen in sarcoidosis or the Guillain Barré Syndrome (idiopathic polyneuritis) or posterior cranial fossa tumours. The rare Melkersson-Rosenthal Syndrome is a condition comprising tongue fissuring, unilateral facial palsy and facial swelling. The lesions are histologically similar to those of Crohn's Disease.

A summary of other cranial nerve lesions is given in *Table 4*. Nerves may be affected by a systemic cause eg diabetes mellitus, MS or there may be a local cause. Multiple cranial nerve palsies may occur in Bulbar Palsy that comprises palsy of the tongue, muscles of chewing/swallowing and facial muscles due to loss of function of motor nuclei in the brainstem. The onset may be acute eg in infection such as polio, or may be chronic eg in tumours of the posterior cranial fossa.

Tics or involuntary facial movements may occasionally be seen in patients. These may be habitual, particularly in children or may be drug induced or they may have a more organic cause. Drug induced dyskinesias are common in the elderly on long-term phenothiazine (antipsychotic) medication which is usually reversible on stopping the drug. Intracranial nerve compression may result in blepharospasm (contraction of both eyelids). Hemifacial muscle spasm may occur and suggests a lesion eg of the cerebello-pontine angle compressing the facial nerve. Whenever a facial tic is found, consideration should be given to referral for investigation since an underlying cause may often be treated.

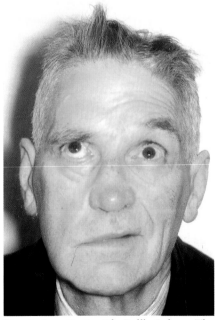

Fig. 1 A patient with Bell's Palsy. The ipsilateral forehead affected also indicating a lower motor neurone lesion. Bell's sign (see text) is also demonstrated

Table 3 Some possible causes of facial weakness (mostly unilateral)		
Idiopathic	-	Bell's Palsy Melkersson-Rosenthal Syndrome
Infection	-	Ear infections TB Ramsay Hunt Syndrome Glandular Fever AIDS
Trauma	-	Facial lacerations/bruising in the region of the facial nerve Penetrating parotid injuries Post-parotid surgery
Neoplastic	-	Primary or secondary cancers Neuroma of facial nerve Acoustic neuroma
Metabolic	-	Diabetes Mellitus Pregnancy Sarcoidosis Guillain-Barré Syndrome

In the **Ramsay-Hunt Syndrome**, a profound facial paralysis is accompanied by vesicles in the pharynx on the same side and in the external auditory meatus. It is thought that the geniculate ganglion of the facial nerve is infected with herpes zoster.

Infections affecting the nervous system may be bacterial or viral in origin. The possibility of bacterial meningitis should be borne in mind with maxillofacial injuries involving the middle third of the face. Prompt treatment with antimicrobials (prophylactically in trauma cases) should be undertaken. The viral type of meningitis is usually mild and self-limiting. The patient with meningitis has a severe headache, feels sick or actively vomits and is often drowsy. The painful, stiff neck and aversion to light are well known. In meningitis caused by the bacterium *Neisseria meningitidis*, a purpuric rash may be seen on the skin and can progress to adrenocortical failure as a result of bleeding into the adrenal cortex.

Herpetic encephalitis is rare, but should be treated promptly with aciclovir. In HIV associated neurological disease, a wide variety of infections

and tumours are seen, for example lymphomas. Neurological effects of such lesions vary from fits to limb weakness.

Brain abscess is a condition that may be secondary to oral sepsis[6] or infection elsewhere eg the middle ear or paranasal sinuses. A patient with congenital heart disease is also at increased risk. Such abscesses can be a complication of infective endocarditis which should be specifically asked about. Signs and symptoms resulting from a brain abscess depend on its location and CT and MRI scanning are useful in localisation and diagnosis. Urgent surgical drainage is required.

Cerebral Palsy is primarily a disorder of motor function secondary to cerebral damage, most frequently associated with birth injury or hypoxia. It is the most common cause of a congenital physical handicap, the patterns of which are variable. There are three main subtypes - spastic, ataxic and athetoid varieties. In the spastic type the muscles are contracted and there may be associated epilepsy. In the ataxic type, a cerebellar lesion is responsible for a disturbance of balance. Writhing movements characterise the athetoid type of cerebral palsy.

In **spina bifida**, the vertebral arches fail to fuse, possibly due to a deficiency of folic acid during foetal development. The condition may lead to significant physical handicap such as an inability to walk, epilepsy or learning difficulties. There may be an association with hydrocephalus which often requires decompression using a shunt. This is discussed further in Chapter 10.

Patients with **syringomyelia** have a condition in which cavitation of the central spinal cord occurs leading to a loss in pain and temperature sensibility. Syringobulbia is the term used if the brain stem is affected - facial sensory loss may occur, as may tongue weakness.

An **acoustic neuroma** is a benign tumour occurring at the cerebellopontine angle on the vestibular part of the vestibulocochlear nerve. Cranial

nerves V, VII, IX and X may also be involved leading to tinnitus, deafness and vertigo. Facial twitching weakness or paraesthesias may occur. Other causes of facial sensory loss (innervated by the trigeminal nerve except over the angle of the mandible which is innervated by cervical nerves) are given in *Table 5*.

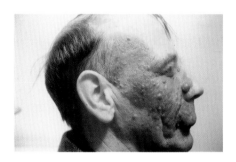

Fig. 2 A patient with Sturge Weber Syndrome

Other neurological disorders that may be encountered include **Huntington's Chorea**, which is an autosomal dominant disorder where there is progressive dementia with marked involuntary movements. The signs do not begin to appear until middle age. **Friedreich's Ataxia** is an autosomal recessive or sometimes sex-linked cord degeneration of unknown cause. Severe ataxia and deformity occurs and there may be associated cardiac disease with arrhythmias.

GENERAL EXAMINATION

The patient's gait may give an immediate clue to an underlying neurological condition, for example the shuffling gait of Parkinsonism. A spastic gait is demonstrated by stiff limbs that are often swung around in a circular motion as the forward movement proceeds.

The patient with a neurological condition may appear confused. This may be for several reasons and a summary of potential causes is given in *Table 6*. Raised intracranial pressure can occur following trauma to the head for example in a patient attending with an injury associated with dental trauma. Such patients will complain of headache and may be restless or vomiting.

Table 4 Cranial Nerve Dysfunction and signs arising from it.		
Cranial nerve	Possible problem	Sign
I Olfactory	Trauma, tumour	Decreased ability to smell
II Optic	Trauma, tumour MS, stroke	Blindness, visual field defect
III Oculomotor	Diabetes, increased intra-cranial pressure	Dilated pupil Ptosis
IV Trochlear	Trauma	Diplopia
V Trigeminal	Sensory - idiopathic, Trauma, IDN/Lingual damage Motor - Bulbar palsy Acoustic Neuroma	None, sensory deficit on testing Signs in IX, X, XI, XII May be decreased facial sensation. Affects VIII also
VI Abducens	MS, some strokes	Inability of eye to look laterally Eye deviated towards nose
VII Facial	LMN – Lower motor neurone Bell's Palsy, skull fracture parotid tumour UMN – Upper motor neurone Stroke, tumour	Total facial weakness Forehead sparing weakness
VIII Vestibulo-Cochlear	Excess noise; Paget's, acoustic neuroma	Deafness
IX Glosso-pharyngeal	Trauma, tumour	Impaired gag reflex
X Vagus	Trauma, brainstem lesions	Impaired gag reflex Soft palate moves to 'good' side on saying 'aah'.
XI Accessory	Polio, stroke	Weakness turning head away from affected side (sternocleidomastoid). Weakness shrugging shoulders (trapezius)
XII Hypoglossal	Trauma, brainstem Lesions	Tongue deviated to affected side on protrusion

The classical sign of increased blood pressure and decreased pulse rate occur and there is dilation of the pupil on the same side as the lesion. Patients with a head injury can be assessed according to the **Glasgow Coma Scale (GCS)** which involves three scored categories of assessment – eye opening, muscle responses and responses to vocal stimuli.

Horner's Syndrome comprises the four signs of a constricted pupil, ptosis (drooping of the upper eyelid), loss of sweating on the ipsilateral face and enophthalmos. It is caused by interference with the cervical sympathetic chain eg after a radical neck dissection, trauma to the neck or tumour.

Patients with cerebral palsy have an increased incidence of dental malocclusion and abnormal movement of the oral and facial musculature that may cause difficulty in dental treatment provision.

The **Sturge-Weber syndrome** (*Fig. 2*) describes an association between a facial port wine stain (haemangioma) with focal fits on the contralateral side. Exophthalmos and spasticity may also be evident. The fits are caused by a capillary haemangioma in the brain.

CONSIDERATION OF THE CRANIAL NERVES

A systematic approach is needed for examining the **Cranial Nerves**. One approach is to consider the cranial nerves in the following groups: ie nerve(s) subserving the sense of smell, eyes, face, mouth, neck and ears. A summary of disorders affecting the cranial nerves and resulting signs is given in *Table 4*.

Any changes in the sense of smell may reflect a problem with the olfactory nerve. Colds and sinusitis may be the cause but trauma involving the cribriform plate can also cause the nerve to have impaired function. Some operations on the nose may cause injury to the olfactory nerves.

Visual acuity may be roughly assessed by asking the patient to read a printed page. Defects of the optic nerve may also affect the field of vision. A lesion of cranial nerve III leads to complete or partial ptosis (drooping of the upper eyelid). The external ocular muscles are controlled by the action of cranial nerves III, IV and VI. Disruption of the third nerve (which supplies all of the extrinsic eye muscles apart from superior oblique and lateral rectus) causes a paralysis of internal, upward and downward movement of the eye leading to double vision. The eye points downwards and outwards except when looking to the affected side. A fixed dilated pupil may also be seen. Disruption of IV, the trochlear nerve supplying superior oblique, prevents the eye moving downwards and medially. The double vision is worse on looking down. Disruption of VI (abducens supplying lateral rectus) causes an inability to abduct the eye (look to the ipsilateral side). There is deviation of the eye towards the nose and double vision.

The muscles of facial expression are innervated by the VII cranial nerve (**facial nerve**). As mentioned previously, upper motor neurone lesions affecting the facial nerve eg after a stroke may be differentiated from lower motor neurone causes eg Bell's Palsy since the latter causes the whole side of the face to be weakened whereas the forehead is spared in an

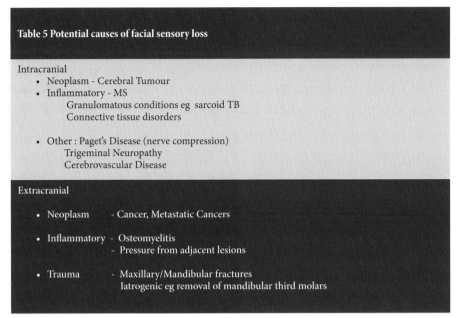

Table 5 Potential causes of facial sensory loss
Intracranial
• Neoplasm - Cerebral Tumour
• Inflammatory - MS
Granulomatous conditions eg sarcoid TB
Connective tissue disorders
• Other : Paget's Disease (nerve compression)
Trigeminal Neuropathy
Cerebrovascular Disease
Extracranial
• Neoplasm   - Cancer, Metastatic Cancers
• Inflammatory - Osteomyelitis
- Pressure from adjacent lesions
• Trauma   - Maxillary/Mandibular fractures
Iatrogenic eg removal of mandibular third molars

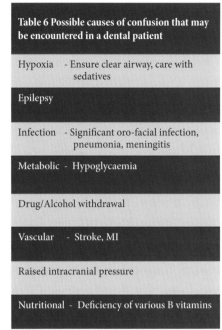

Table 6 Possible causes of confusion that may be encountered in a dental patient	
Hypoxia	- Ensure clear airway, care with sedatives
Epilepsy	
Infection	- Significant oro-facial infection, pneumonia, meningitis
Metabolic	- Hypoglycaemia
Drug/Alcohol withdrawal	
Vascular	- Stroke, MI
Raised intracranial pressure	
Nutritional	- Deficiency of various B vitamins

upper motor neurone lesion due to bilateral representation at the level of the cerebral cortex. The ipsilateral eye moves upwards on attempted closure of the eyes in Bell's Palsy – this is known as Bell's Sign (*Fig. 1*).

In terms of **facial sensation** the sensory division of the trigeminal (V cranial) nerve subserves this over most of the face. The ophthalmic, maxillary and mandibular divisions may be compared by testing skin sensation on either side with a wisp of cotton wool. The corneal (blink) reflex is often the first clinical deficit to be seen in trigeminal nerve lesions.

The **mouth** can demonstrate signs of cranial nerve problems in the case of cranial nerves V (motor division), IX, X and XII. If the masseter muscles are palpated whilst asking the patient to clench the teeth and the motor division of V is inactive, the masseter on that side will not contract properly. With a unilateral lesion, the mandible deviates to the weak side on opening the mouth (V being motor to the pterygoid muscles).

Asking the patient to say 'aah' will allow an appraisal of IX and X nerves. The ninth (glossopharyngeal) nerve is mainly sensory for the pharynx and palate and the tenth (vagus) mainly motor. With a unilateral lesion of the vagus, the soft palate is pulled away from the weaker side. Lesions of both nerves lead to an impaired gag reflex. The twelfth (hypoglossal) nerve may

be tested by asking the patient to protrude the tongue. The tongue deviates to the weaker side.

To test the accessory (eleventh) cranial nerve the patient should be asked to put their chin towards the left or right shoulder against resistance by the examiner. The sternomastoid muscle (supplied by XI) does not function when XI is affected.

The **eighth** (**vestibulocochlear**) nerve has two components - the vestibular (appreciation of position and movements of the head) and the cochlear (responsible for hearing). Lesions of the nerve may cause hearing loss, vertigo or ringing in the ears (tinnitus). Special tests are needed to test the balance and positional functions of the nerve.

GENERAL AND LOCAL ANAESTHESIA, SEDATION AND MANAGEMENT CONSIDERATIONS IN THE DENTAL PATIENT WITH NEUROLOGICAL DISEASE

Patients prone to syncope should be treated with regard to avoidance of known precipitating factors as far as possible. Treatment in the supine position has obvious advantages.

Epileptic patients referred for GA should not be given methohexitone or enflurane since these are epileptogenic. It is important to ensure that an epileptic patient has taken their normal medication on the day of the procedure. Intravenous sedation is useful

in managing epileptic patients. The benzodiazepines have anticonvulsant properties and anxiolysis should decrease the chances of a fit. When treating epileptic patients with sedation supplemental oxygen should be provided via a nasal cannula.[7] The use of the benzodiazepine reversal agent flumazenil should be avoided in patients with epilepsy as this drug can precipitate convulsions.

Patients who have had a CVA should have treatment if possible only when their condition has been optimised. There may be a loss of reflexes such as swallowing or the gag reflex, which has implications for the safe provision of treatment under LA, with or without sedation. Ability to protect the airway is also relevant for the provision of GA since all these modes of treatment jeopardise the airway to some extent. Stroke patients may be taking anticoagulants, or may be hypertensive.

In both multiple sclerosis and motor neurone disease, the degree of compliance achievable for treatment is likely to be impaired. It is best to use LA alone if possible. Limited mobility and/or associated psychological disorders may cause difficulties with treatment. Patients are better treated sitting so that respiration is assisted as much as possible since it may be impaired. Patients with MS may be taking corticosteroids, particularly early in the disease. Care of the airway may be made more difficult due to muscular incoordination.

Patients with Parkinson's disease suffer from excess salivation, which can cause difficulties with visibility not only in providing the treatment itself but also for the safe provision of an anaesthetic. Anti-muscarinic drugs will reduce the salivation and degree of tremor. The autonomic insufficiency often found in these patients makes them liable to postural hypotension and poor candidates for GA.

In myasthenia gravis, local anaesthetic is the option of choice. Doses should be kept to a minimum. Muscle fatigue appears to increase during the day and therefore treatment is best carried out early. Intravenous sedation should not be given in a dental practice setting[8] since respiratory impairment may be worsened. A small oral dose of a benzodiazepine is acceptable if the patient is very anxious about their treatment. For similar reasons general anaesthetics are also not advised if possible. In addition, some of the agents used with GA eg the muscle relaxant suxamethonium or opioids eg fentanyl may have their effects potentiated in these patients.

Patients with problems with vision may be permanently disabled or the disorder may be transient. It is important that a 'tell-do' approach is used for these patients to minimise anxiety. It is worth bearing in mind in these patients that other senses eg hearing may be heightened. Diplopia can be a transient complication of LA as mentioned earlier. Other cranial nerve lesions of potential relevance include lesions affecting cranial nerves IX and X since the gag reflex may be impaired leading to potential airway compromise, particularly if sedation or GA are being used.

Patients with cerebral palsy may not be able to tolerate treatment under LA and GA may be the only way of achieving it. In the athetoid type, potential epilepsy should be borne in mind. Anxiety will often worsen the effects of the cerebral palsy and therefore premedication eg with diazepam is often wise. Patients with spina bifida have increased incidence of latex allergy. Such patients may be prone to postural hypotension and are therefore best treated sitting up. Epilepsy and renal anomalies may also be associated. In Friedreich's Ataxia, possible arrhythmias should be remembered.

EFFECTS OF DRUGS USED IN NEUROLOGICAL DISORDERS ON ORO-DENTAL STRUCTURES

Drugs used to treat neurological conditions can produce unwanted effects in and around the mouth. Anticonvulsants have a number of unwanted effects of interest to dentists. Gingival overgrowth is a recognised side effect of phenytoin[9] but may also occur with sodium valproate and ethosuximide. In addition, phenytoin causes taste disturbance and may produce Stevens-Johnson syndrome. This drug may also affect the teeth. It has been implicated in producing hypercementosis and shortening of the roots.[10] Sodium valproate may produce parotid gland enlargement. Lamotrigine may cause dry mouth and Stevens-Johnson syndrome. Ethosuximide may produce Stevens Johnson syndrome and gingival bleeding. Carbamazepine may produce xerostomia, glossitis and oral ulceration. Stevens-Johnson syndrome is the name given to a severe form of erythema multiforme. The latter predominantly affects young males and is characterized by mucosal lesions with or without skin lesions. The typical skin lesion is described as looking like a target as it consists of concentric erythematous rings. The rashes may appear differently however, hence the name 'multiforme'. The aetiology of erythema multiforme is not known but is thought to be a disorder of immune complexes. The antigens can be as diverse as microorganisms or drugs.

The anti-muscarinic anti-Parkinsonian drugs such as orphenadrine and benzhexol can produce dry mouth, which may increase caries incidence. In addition, the dopaminergics drugs such as levodopa and co-careldopa may produce taste disturbances.

SUMMARY

As with disorders of other systems, neurological diseases impact on dental treatment provision, both in terms of the treatment itself and the provision of safe methods of anaesthesia/analgesia to facilitate it.

1. Divya K S, Moran N A, Atkin P A. Numb chin syndrome: a case series and discussion. *Br Dent J* 2010; **208:** 157-60.
2. Talukdar B, Chakrabarty B. Efficacy of buccal midazolam compared to intravenous diazepam in controlling convulsions in children: a randomized controlled trial. *Brain Dev* 2009; **31:** 744-9.
3. Madland G, Newton-John T, Feinmann C. Chronic idiopathic Orofacial pain: I: What is the evidence base? *Br Dent J* 2001; **191:** 22 – 24.
4. Nurmikko T J, Eldridge P R. Trigeminal neuralgia – pathophysiology, diagnosis and current treatment. *Br J Anaesth* 2001; **87:** 117 – 132.
5. Courtney D J, Thomas S, Whitfield P H. Isolated orbital blowout fractures: survey and review. *Br J Oral Maxillofac Surg* 2000; **38:** 496 – 502.
6. Corson M A, Postlethwaite K R, Seymour R A. Are dental infections a cause of brain abscess? Case report and review of the literature. *Oral Diseases* 2001, **7:** 61-65.
7. Meechan J G, Robb N D, Seymour R A. *Pain and Anxiety Control for the Conscious Dental Patient.* pp 287 – 290. Oxford, Oxford University Press, 1998.
8. Malamed S F. *Sedation: a Guide to Patient Management 3rd ed.* p595 – 596. St Louis: Mosby, 1995.
9. Hassell T M. *Epilepsy and the Oral Manifestations of Phenytoin Therapy.* Basle: Kruger, 1981.
10. Seymour R A, Meechan J G, Walton J G. *Adverse Drug Reactions in Dentistry 2nd ed.* p 121. Oxford: Oxford University Press, 1996.

Chapter 5
Liver disease

M. Greenwood and J. G. Meechan

IN BRIEF
- Liver disorders are important to the dentist due to a potential bleeding tendency, intolerance to drugs eg general anaesthetics, benzodiazepines and the possibility of underlying infective causes for the liver dysfunction.
- Signs of liver disease include jaundice, spider naevi, leuconychia, finger clubbing, palmar erythema, Dupuytren's contracture, sialosis and gynaecomastia.
- The general anaesthetic agent halothane (now used infrequently) should not be given twice to the same patient within 3 months. A 'halothane hepatitis' is likely to result.
- Dental sedation should only be performed in specialist units for patients with significant liver disease as small doses can lead to coma.

The liver has a number of important functions. It metabolises drugs and endogenous substances and contributes to their excretion by the body. Plasma proteins are synthesised in the liver which also acts as a storage organ for glycogen and vitamin B_{12}. The liver is also important in the production of clotting factors for normal haemostatic function.

POINTS IN THE HISTORY

The history may reveal evidence of liver disease. This is important in terms of potential **drug toxicity**, **bleeding tendency** and the possibility of **viral hepatitis**. Chronic liver disease (defined as liver disease present for more than 6 months) can enter an acute phase if unrecognised eg after the administration of sedation. Acute liver failure itself may be precipitated

Table 1 Serological markers for Hepatitis B

Hepatitis B Surface Antigen - first manifestion of infection
Antibody to Hepatitis B Surface Antigen - associated with protection from infection
Hepatitis B Core Antigen - detected by development of antibody and signifies donor infectivity if surface antigen negative but core antigen positive
Hepatitis B e Antigen - only found if HBs Antigen positive (an index of infectivity)

by any type of viral hepatitis, the anaesthetic agent halothane, paracetamol overdose or Reye's Syndrome (see later).

Viral hepatitis is clearly of importance to the dentist.[1] Indeed, dental students must show satisfactory immunisation against hepatitis B in order to undergo clinical training in the United Kingdom.[2] **Hepatitis A** is transmitted via the faeco-oral route and has a 3-week incubation period. There is no known carrier state. **Hepatitis B** may be transmitted by blood to blood contact eg via contaminated sharps, and droplet infection. It has an incubation period of 6 weeks to 6 months. A small proportion of patients will progress to a hepatitis B carrier state associated with chronic active hepatitis and eventually cirrhosis. The presence of Hepatitis B Surface Antigen (HBsAg) is the first manifestation of infection. The presence of antibody to HBs is associated

with protection from infection. Hepatitis B Core Antigen (HBcAg) is detected by the development of an antibody to it. It may persist for 1 to 2 years signifying donor infectivity if HBsAg negative but HBcAg positive. Hepatitis B e Antigen is only found in HBsAg positive sera and appears during the incubation period. It is an index of infectivity. DNA polymerase is first detected when the level of HBsAg is increasing, and indicates the presence of virions in the serum and is associated with replication. A summary of serological markers for hepatitis B is given in *Table 1*.

Hepatitis C can be contracted from a contaminated blood transfusion. **Hepatitis D** (or delta) is a viral RNA associated with hepatitis B and demonstrated in association with HBcAg. Other viral causes of a hepatitis include Cytomegalovirus, Herpes Simplex, Epstein Barr Virus and Coxsackie B Virus.

Efficient cross infection control[3] should minimise the risk of contracting the infective types of hepatitis. There is an adjunct in the form of a **hepatitis B vaccine** (Engerix B). This vaccine is injected into the deltoid muscle of the upper arm and is repeated at 1 and 6 months after the original dose. Serology is used to time boosters and identify none or poor responders. Poor responders tend to be members of the older population, smokers and male. An anti-HBs level of less than one hundred is not enough to confer protection and in such cases a booster is required and a further level checked a month later. Even with a good response it is not until 6 weeks after the first injection that protection is achieved and therefore a specific anti-hepatitis B immunoglobulin is required for individuals exposed to the virus during this time.

A history of *jaundice* may be obtained. This does not necessarily imply liver disease eg bile duct obstruction due to gallstones or malignant disease may also cause jaundice. Jaundice at birth is common and is usually of no significance. Normally, bilirubin (a breakdown product of haemoglobin) is conjugated in the liver where it becomes water soluble and is excreted in the bile which colours the faeces. If the bilirubin is not conjugated eg due to parenchymal liver disease, it colours the skin and mucous membrane ('jaundice'). In obstructive jaundice, bile does not reach the gut leading to pale faeces but there is increased urinary bilirubin, the urine therefore is dark. Dark urine and pale faeces are a hallmark of obstructive jaundice.

It is important to suspect and enquire about any *bleeding tendency* (and testing of clotting is required). Poor absorption of fat soluble vitamin K occurs with its attendant effects on clotting and there is also decreased synthesis of clotting factors.

Obstruction to blood flow in the liver (portal circulation) leads to an increase in portal blood pressure with formation of enlarged blood vessels (varices) at the base of the oesophagus (one place where systemic and portal circulations meet) with consequent risk of gastrointestinal haemorrhage. Chronic bleeding may lead to anaemia.

In **cirrhosis** of the liver, the architecture is irreversibly destroyed by fibrosis and regenerating nodules of hepatocytes. The cause is often unknown but a quarter of cases are alcohol related. Hepatitis B or C, and the chemotherapy drug methotrexate can all be implicated. Primary biliary cirrhosis (PBC) is a disease primarily of females thought to be autoimmune in origin. It can be associated with Sjogren's Syndrome or oral lichen planus.[4]

The most common liver tumours are **metastases**. These signal advanced disease and the outlook depends on the extent and nature of the primary tumour. Recent advances in surgery have meant that in certain situations resection of metastases is possible and chemotherapy may be appropriate. Jaundice, if present at all, is a late sign. Hepatocellular cancer may occur after hepatitis B or C infection and cirrhosis of the primary biliary type.

The patient may give a history of liver problems after certain **medications**. Likely to be of interest to the dentist are aspirin, carbamazepine, erythromycin estolate, tetracycline and halothane.[5] Halothane is discussed later. Aspirin is not indicated in children due to the risk of Reye's Syndrome which comprises liver damage and encephalopathy occurring after aspirin ingestion.

Patients may be encountered who have undergone a liver transplant - the most common indication for which is end-stage liver disease. Management considerations are discussed later.

Familial conditions may occur eg Gilbert's Syndrome in which the bilirubin level increases but is not conjugated and therefore does not enter the urine. It generally presents as mild jaundice. Many patients have no symptoms but some have episodes of malaise, anorexia and upper abdominal pain with jaundice. These episodes may be related to infection, fatigue or fasting.

A summary of the main areas of enquiry in a patient with liver disease is given in *Table 2*.

EXAMINATION

There may be significant clues to the presence of liver disease that are discernible from a patient sitting in a dental chair, (*Table 3*).

The hands may show a Dupuytren's contracture (a condition in which the ring and little fingers are held flexed when the hand is held passive due to thickened palmar fascial tissue) or there may be palmar erythema. The fingers may be clubbed, and the fingernails may have a whitish colouration (leuconychia). If the hands are held outstretched in front of the patient a marked flapping tremor may be noted – 'liver flap' in severe liver decompensation.

Oedema (secondary to hypoproteinaemia) may lead to ascites (fluid in the abdomen leading to distension) or ankle oedema. The commonest cause of the latter however is likely to be cardiovascular. Itching may produce scratch marks on the skin. The itching occurs due to deposition of bile salts in the skin. The patient may be jaundiced. Gynaecomastia (enlarged breast tissue in the male) may occur due to increased circulating oestrogen levels. This also said to be responsible for the palmar erythema mentioned earlier. Spider naevi (numerous thin, tortuous blood vessels emanating from a central arteriole) may occur on the face, neck, upper chest and back (said to be within the distribution of the superior vena cava). Parotid enlargement (sialosis)[6] may be seen in cases of cirrhosis but this is due to the associated alcohol intake rather than the cirrhosis itself.

FACTORS AFFECTING DENTAL TREATMENT UNDER GA/LA/ SEDATION

Agents such as sedatives and general anaesthetics can be potentially dangerous in liver disease mainly due to impairment of detoxification. In the case of halothane, a hepatitis may follow its use especially in the obese, in smokers and in middle aged

Table 2 Points in the history in a patient with liver disease

- Hepatitis
- History of jaundice
- Bleeding tendency
- Cirrhosis
- Liver tumours
- Reaction to medications
- Liver surgery eg transplants
- Familial disorders

Table 3 Signs that may be seen in a patient with a chronic liver disorder

- Dupuytren's contracture
- Palmar erythema
- Finger clubbing
- Leuconychia
- Parotid enlargement
- Jaundice
- Spider naevi
- Gynaecomastia
- Ascites/ankle oedema
- Scratch marks (itching)

females and if a halothane anaesthetic has been given in the last 3 months. The precise mechanism is not known. The hepatitis tends to develop after about a week and comprises jaundice, malaise and anorexia. The newer agents eg enflurane, sevoflurane are less hepatotoxic and as a result the use of halothane has waned.

A patient with a history or signs suggestive of a liver disorder or a high alcohol intake which might potentially cause liver damage should have blood taken for liver function tests (LFTs) and clotting studies. These should be carried out prior to GA or surgery. Severe bleeding can occur after dental extractions in patients with chronic liver disease[7] so the clotting status must be tested. There are many different types of LFT but the commonest involve measurement of Aspartate Transaminase (AST) and Alanine Transaminase (ALT). ALT may also be raised in cardiac or skeletal muscle damage and is therefore not specific for liver disease. Gamma Glutamyl Transferase (yGT), when it is raised, usually reflects alcoholic liver disease. Alkaline Phosphatase levels may be raised in obstructive jaundice but this is not a specific marker. The level of alpha fetoprotein may be raised in hepatocellular cancer. In cirrhosis, treatment should only be carried out in conjunction with the patient's physician. Relative analgesia is preferred to sedation with a benzodiazepine. A specialist anaesthetist is required even if GA is acceptable.

In many liver diseases brain metabolism is altered and it therefore becomes more sensitive to certain drugs. Encephalopathy can be triggered by sedatives or opiates. In obstructive jaundice, the main risk is bleeding due to vitamin K malabsorption. If surgery is required in such patients, intravenous vitamin K may be required for several days beforehand to correct any bleeding tendency. Any patient with jaundice has an increased risk of bleeding excessively following any surgical procedure including dental extractions. A peri-operative infusion of fresh frozen plasma will often be required. If the patient is severely jaundiced a GA may precipitate renal failure, the **Hepato-Renal Syndrome**. The risk is decreased if the patient is well hydrated with intravenous fluids and given the osmotic diuretic mannitol to ensure a good urine flow pre, per and post-operatively.

Local anaesthesia is not entirely safe in patients with hepatic impairment. Most of the amide local anaesthetics used in dental practice undergo biotransformation in the liver. Articaine is metabolized partly in plasma[8] and prilocaine receives some metabolism in the lungs.[9] However, the liver is the main site of metabolic activity. All of an injected dose of local anaesthetic will eventually reach the circulation and if metabolism is affected the concentration in plasma will slowly increase. Only about 2% of the drug will be excreted unchanged. This may lead to signs of CNS toxicity with relatively low doses, as little as two cartridges in an adult patient may be too much if liver disease is severe.

If possible a full dental assessment should be carried out prior to a liver transplant particularly since post-operatively the patient will be immunosuppressed. Invasive dental treatment should only be carried out after consultation with the patient's physician. After transplantation no elective dental treatment should be carried out for the first 3 months. GA, if needed, must be carried out in units with the required expertise.

Dental sedation should only be performed in specialist units for patients with significant liver disease as small doses can lead to coma.

PRESCRIBING FOR PATIENTS WITH LIVER DISEASE.

The use of any drug in a patient with severe liver disease should be discussed with the patient's physician. Hepatic impairment will lead to failure of metabolism of many drugs that can result in toxicity. In some cases dose reduction is required, other drugs should be avoided completely.

The British National Formulary[10] lists those drugs that should be avoided or used with caution in patients with liver disease. Dentists should note that the anti-fungal drug miconazole is contra-indicated if there is hepatic impairment and flucanazole requires dose reduction. Erythromycin, metronidazole and tetracyclines should be avoided. Non-steroidal anti-inflammatory drugs increase the risk of gastro-intestinal bleeding and interfere with fluid balance and are best avoided. Paracetamol doses should be reduced as at high doses this drug is hepatotoxic.

SUMMARY

Knowledge of liver disorders is important for the safe delivery of dental care. A thorough history will usually alert the clinician to potential problems. Haemostasis may be affected and this should be particularly borne in mind.

1. Anders P L, Fabiano J P, Thines T J. Hepatitis: still a concern? *Spec Care Dent* 2000; **20:** 209 – 213.
2. Laszlo J, Ivarajasingam V, Ogden G R. A virus, the vice-chancellors and principles of vaccination. *Br Dent J* 1996; **180:** 124 – 126.
3. Infection control in dentistry. BDA advice sheet A12. BDA 2000.
4. Gart G S, Camisa C. Ulcerative and oral lichen planus associated with sicca syndrome and primary biliary cirrhosis. *Cutis* 1994; **53:** 249 – 250.

5. Seymour R A, Meechan J G, Walton J G. *Adverse Drug Reactions in Dentistry 2nd ed.* pp 41 – 42. Oxford: Oxford University Press, 1996.
6. Kastin B, Mandel L. Alcoholic sialosis. *New York Dent J* 2000; **66:** 22 – 24.
7. Thomson P J, Langton S G. Persistent haemorrhage following dental extractions in patients with liver disease: two cautionary tales. *Br Dent J* 1996; **184:** 141 – 144.
8. Jastak J T, Yagiela J A, Donaldson D. *Local Anesthesia of the Oral Cavity.* p 90. Philadelphia: W.B. Saunders, 1995.
9. Jastak J T, Yagiela J A, Donaldson D. *Local Anesthesia of the Oral Cavity.* pp 98 – 100. Philadelphia: W.B. Saunders, 1995.
10. British National Formulary. Online at http:// bnf.org.

Chapter 6
The endocrine system

M. Greenwood and J. G. Meechan

IN BRIEF

- Diabetic patients should be treated first on a treatment session so that the start time is predictable. Hypoglycaemia must be avoided and presents more quickly than hyperglycaemia. A physician should be consulted if a general anaesthetic is being considered.
- Thyroid disease may present as a goitre. Thyroid function should be stabilised before a general anaesthetic is used.
- Oral contraceptives may predispose to thromboembolism and their action may be impaired by some antibiotics and anticonvulsants.
- In pregnancy essential treatment should be carried out in the second trimester when possible.
- Acromegaly may be associated with headaches, visual loss, diabetes and hypertension

The endocrine system consists of glands that produce hormones that may exert their effects at distant sites. Widespread problems may result when there is derangement of the system. Disorders may have a bearing on the management of a dental patient either in terms of the treatment itself or the provision of a specific method of anaesthesia.

POINTS IN THE HISTORY

The patient may suffer from **diabetes mellitus (DM)**. This is a persistent state of hyperglycaemia due to either a lack of insulin or a diminished physiological effect of the hormone after production by the pancreas. DM may be diagnosed by two fasting venous blood glucose levels of greater than or equal to 7.8 millimoles per litre. The disease may be Type I (Insulin Dependent Diabetes Mellitus IDDM) or Type II (Non-insulin Dependent Diabetes Mellitus NIDDM). Type I occurs most frequently in young people, whilst Type II is usually a maturity onset diabetes. Type II diabetes is treated by careful diet or oral hypoglycaemics. Factors predisposing to DM include pancreatic disease and drugs eg thiazide diuretics, steroids. Other endocrine disorders such as Cushing's Disease, phaeochromocytoma and acromegaly (all of which are discussed later) may also be relevant as the likelihood of DM is increased in these disorders. The diabetic tendency tends to resolve if the underlying disorder is corrected.

Good control of DM helps to prevent or manage some of the associated complications of the disease which particularly relate to the cardiovascular system and retina. DM may be asymptomatic, but the patient may have noticed drinking excessive fluids, passing lots of urine, lethargy, weight loss and possibly recurrent skin infections.

It is important to ascertain some idea of the degree of diabetic control - patients will often know their typical blood sugar level and have experienced episodes of hypoglycaemia or 'hypo's', which is discussed in more detail later.

Abnormalities of the circulating level of thyroxine are usually due to disorders of the **thyroid gland** and may be due to over production (hyperthyroidism) or under production (hypothyroidism). Two main hormones are produced by the thyroid gland - T3 (tri-iodothyronine) and T4 (thyroxine) - the former is five times as active as the latter, and both are bound to protein in the blood. The hypothalamus produces Thyroid Releasing Hormone (TRH) stimulating the release of Thyroid Stimulating Hormone (TSH) from the anterior pituitary, which in turn causes release of T3 and T4 from the thyroid. Details of hyper and hypothyroidism are given in *Table 1*, and the pathway of T3 and T4 production in *Fig. 1*. Hypothyroidism may decrease the immune response leading to an increased incidence of opportunistic infections such as oral candidosis.

Many patients will be taking the **oral contraceptive pill (OCP)** which comprises varying proportions of synthetic oestrogens and progestogens. It is the oestrogen component that tends to cause complications. The major risk is the increased risk of thromboembolic disease, especially deep vein thrombosis (DVT). Hypertension and a diabetic tendency are other potential risks. The 'pill' is usually maintained for minor procedures but if a prolonged GA is being given, prophylaxis against DVT eg subcutaneous heparin, should be given due to the increased risk from venous stasis. Some surgeons would recommend discontinuing the OCP for two months prior to a surgical procedure to eliminate the potential for the complications mentioned above.

Many patients are receiving **Hormone Replacement Therapy** (**HRT**) which may be given orally or as an implant and aims to replace oestrogen which is deficient due to reduced secretion eg after the menopause or ovary removal. Osteoporosis is inhibited in the patient on HRT and it also appears to reduce the rate of alveolar bone resorption.

A patient may be unaware of **pregnancy**, especially in the first two months, a time when the foetus is particularly vulnerable. In diabetic patients good control of blood sugar levels may become more difficult during pregnancy. Diabetes may occur for the first time in pregnancy (gestational diabetes) and this usually resolves after birth. In the later stages the patient should not be laid fully supine since the gravid uterus compresses the inferior vena cava and impedes venous return. Likewise, in the unlikely event of having to carry out CPR on a pregnant patient, it is important that the patient is put in a left lateral position otherwise venous return would be similarly impeded.

Cardiac output is increased in pregnancy which leads to a tachycardia. Hypertension in pregnancy will often be asymptomatic but should always be taken seriously. If the hypertension is associated with protein in the urine and oedema the condition is known as pre-eclampsia. This may culminate in eclampsia (hypertension, protein in urine and convulsions) and can have fatal consequences.

Cushing's Disease occurs as a result of excess glucocorticoid production secondary to adrenal hyperplasia. The adrenal hyperplasia, in turn may be secondary to excess adrenocorticotrophic hormone (ACTH) production eg by a pituitary adenoma. Ectopic ACTH may be produced by a small cell lung cancer, producing similar

Table 1 Hyperthyroidism and hypothyroidism

	Hyperthyroidism	Hypothyroidism
Causes:	Grave's Disease - Antibodies against TSH receptors. Common cause in women between 30-50 years. Other causes: Toxic multinodular goitre, some thyroid cancers.	Spontaneous - Primary Atrophic Drug induced eg Antithyroid drugs Iodine deficiency
Symptoms:	Weight loss Dislike of heat Tremor, irritability Emotionally labile	Weight gain Dislike of cold Lethargy Depression
Signs:	Tachycardia Atrial fibrillation Tremor Enlarged thyroid Exophthalmos Diplopia	Bradycardia Goitre Dry skin and hair
Treatment:	Carbimazole Partial Thyroidectomy Radioactive Iodine	Thyroxine replacement

effects. The hypothalamo-pituitary-adrenal axis is shown in *Fig. 2*.

Cushing's Syndrome is similar clinically, but caused by primary adrenal disease eg cancer or adenoma. The terms Cushing's Syndrome and Cushing's Disease are often used synonymously – but incorrectly. The clinical features are discussed later.

Patients with **Conn's Syndrome** have a tumour or hyperplasia of the adrenal cortex. The resulting high levels of aldosterone secretion lead to potassium loss and sodium retention. The decreased potassium leads to muscle weakness and polyuria, whereas sodium retention leads to hypertension.

Addison's Disease is a disease of the adrenal glands leading to decreased secretion of cortisol and aldosterone. The cause may be tuberculous destruction of the adrenals but is not known in up to 80% of cases. There may be an association with Grave's Disease (see later) or IDDM. If known, the cause is treated but replacement steroids are needed and a steroid boost is therefore required for surgical dental treatment.

Disorders of the parathyroid glands may occur. The function of parathyroid hormone (PTH), secreted by the glands, is to regulate the level of calcium in the plasma by acting on the kidney, gut and bone. Secretion of

PTH is stimulated if the plasma calcium level falls. The hormone causes increased reabsorption of calcium by the kidney and gut and induces resorption of bone, to restore the calcium level. Hypoparathyroidism occurs most commonly after thyroid surgery since the thyroid and parathyroid glands are anatomically very close (the four parathyroid glands normally lying posterior to the thyroid gland).

Hyperparathyroidism may be classified as primary, secondary or tertiary. The most common cause of primary hyperparathyroidism is a parathyroid gland adenoma. Secondary hyperparathyroidism occurs when there is a chronically low plasma calcium level eg in chronic renal failure or malabsorption. Tertiary hyperparathyroidism is said to occur when the parathyroid glands have started to produce PTH autonomously, usually after a prolonged period of secondary hyperparathyroidism. Hyperparathyroidism may lead to a loss of lamina dura around the teeth and central giant cell granulomas may occur.[1] These are known as brown tumours and are histologically indistinct from other giant cell lesions. If such granulomas are found it is therefore prudent to arrange for a test of calcium and PTH levels.

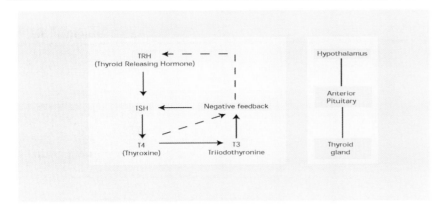

Fig. 1 Production of T3 and T4 in the Thyroid Gland

Table 2 Points in the history in a dental patient with an endocrine disorder

- Diabetes mellitus
    - Insulin dependent
    - Diet or tablet controlled
    - Degree of control achieved

- Thyroid disease
    - Hyper
    - Hypo

- Oral contraceptives

- Pregnancy

- Cushing's disease

- Addison's disease

- Hyper/hypo parathyroidism

- Conn's Syndrome

- History of phaeochromocytoma

- Diabetes insipidus

- Acromegaly

A **phaeochromocytoma** is a rare cause of hypertension. It is a usually benign tumour of the adrenal medulla (usually unilateral) producing excess catecholamines eg adrenaline. Symptoms are episodic and consist of headaches, palpitations and sweating together with pallor and hypertension. Elective treatment should be delayed until the tumour has been dealt with (local anaesthetic injections with epinephrine [adrenaline] should be avoided). Treatment of phaeochromocytoma is surgical and both alpha and beta blockers are used to prevent hypertensive crises during such surgery.

The patient may report having been diagnosed with **Diabetes insipidus** - a condition in which impaired water reabsorption occurs in the kidney either as a result of too little anti-diuretic hormone (ADH) being produced by the posterior pituitary or an impaired response to ADH by the kidney. The patient will complain of drinking lots of fluid and passing lots of urine. Causes include head injury, pituitary tumour or sarcoid. Patients may complain of a dry mouth. The **Syndrome of Inappropriate ADH secretion** (SIADH) may occur secondary to some malignancies and certain benign chest disorders eg pneumonia. It may occur secondary to trauma and is characterised by a low blood sodium level with a high urinary sodium concentration.

Acromegaly (*Fig. 3*) is caused by increased secretion of growth hormone from a pituitary tumour. It has an insidious onset and the clinical features are discussed in the Examination

Section. Relevant complications include hypertension, DM and cardiomyopathy (disease of the cardiac muscle).

The main pancreatic problem of relevance in an endocrine context is DM and is discussed above. Hormone secreting **pancreatic tumours** are rare and include the Zollinger-Ellison Syndrome in which a gastrin secreting tumour leads to duodenal ulceration and diarrhoea. Insulinomas may also occur leading to hypoglycaemia. Glucagonoma leads to hyperglycaemia, oral bullae and erosions.

Nelson's Syndrome affects people who have had bilateral adrenalectomy eg to treat Cushing's Syndrome, which leads to increased pituitary activity and adenoma formation. ACTH is released in great quantities and cutaneous or oral pigmentation may result.

A summary of the main points in the endocrine history is given in *Table 2*.

EXAMINATION OF PATIENTS WITH ENDOCRINE DISORDERS

The diabetic patient may have little or nothing of note to see on clinical examination that gives a clue to their condition. There may be sialosis (swelling of the salivary glands). If diabetic control is poor, oral candidosis may develop. These patients are

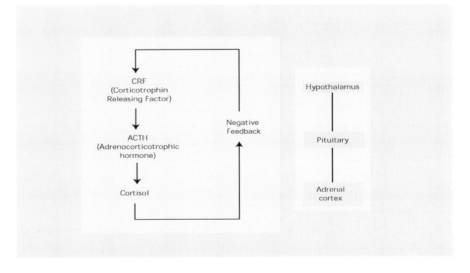

Fig. 2 The hypothalamus-pituitary-adrenal axis

generally more prone to infections and may have more severe gingivitis than might be expected from the level of oral hygiene. Certainly, diabetic patients are more prone to periodontal breakdown compared to healthy patients.[2] The skin is more prone to infections. Peripheral neuropathy may lead to severe foot infections since foreign bodies can be trodden on and not noticed

A **goitre** may be noted. This is a lump in the neck comprising an enlarged thyroid gland, usually due to hyperplasia caused by stimulation by TSH, secondary to a decreased level of circulating thyroid hormone. The thyroid gland begins its development at the foramen caecum at the junction of the posterior one third with the anterior two thirds of the tongue and descends to its normal position in the neck during development. On rare occasions remnants of thyroid tissue remain along the developmental path and may be seen as a lump in the midline lying at any point between foramen caecum and epiglottis, the so-called thyroglossal cyst. A goitre may lead to difficulty in swallowing or even compromise the airway. Thyroid tissue may occasionally be present within the tongue – the so-called 'lingual thyroid'. All goitres should be fully investigated, particularly to exclude cancers.

The poorly controlled hyperthyroid patient is tachycardic and may well be in atrial fibrillation with an irregularly irregular pulse. A fine tremor is sometimes noted and the patient may have exophthalmos with resultant diplopia. The thyroid gland itself may be enlarged. The hypothyroid patient may have a bradycardia, dry skin and hair and a goitre.

A patient with hypoparathyroidism, the commonest cause of which is as a complication of thyroid surgery, may exhibit facial paraesthesia and facial twitching when the preauricular skin over the facial nerve is tapped - known as **Chvostek's Sign**, due to decreased plasma calcium levels.

In a **Cushingoid patient** the tissues are wasted, leading to peripheral myopathy and thin skin which bruises

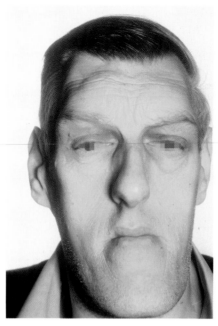

Fig. 3 A patient with acromegaly exhibiting the classic facial appearance

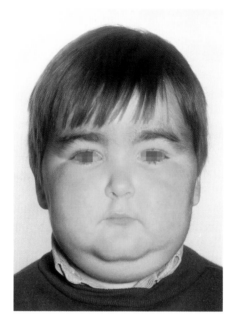

Fig. 4 The facial appearance of a patient taking long-term steroids

easily. Purple striae on the skin (usually abdominal) may also occur. Water retention leads to the characteristic moon face with hypertension and oedema (*Fig. 4*). There is obesity of the trunk, head and neck (buffalo hump). A summary of the clinical features of Cushing's Syndrome is given in *Table 3*. In hypofunction (**Addison's Disease**) hyperpigmentation may be seen eg of palmar creases and buccal mucosa. This pigmentation is related to high circulating

Table 3 The clinical findings in a patient with Cushing's Syndrome
• Moon face • Buffalo hump (excess interscapular fat) • Excess fat on trunk (relative sparing of limbs) • Purple skin striae • Hirsutism • Tendency to acne • Hypertension • Diabetic tendency • Osteoporosis • Peripheral muscle weakness

Table 4 Hypoglycaemia and treatment
Symptoms of Hypoglycaemia Autonomic

- Sweating
- Tremor
- Hunger

Secondary to depressed levels of glucose on nerves

- Drowsy, confused
- Fits
- Perioral tingling
- Loss of consciousness

Treatment in Dental Surgery
Conscious - Oral sugar, 2 teaspoons
Unconscious - 20ml of 50% dextrose IV or 1mg glucagon subcutaneously
Oral glucose when conscious

Table 5 Hyperglycaemia
• Slower onset than hypoglycaemia • Unlikely presentation in a dental surgery • Mainstay of treatment is rehydration

levels of Melanocyte Stimulating Hormone (MSH).

Hirsutism is sometimes seen in Cushing's Syndrome and hyperthyroidism as well as acromegaly. It may also be seen in ovarian or adrenal tumours.

Facial flushing may be seen in phaeochromocytoma due to the release of sympathomimetic substances or may be a sign of the Carcinoid Syndrome due to the over production of 5-hydroxytryptamine. Diarrhoea may be associated with the carcinoid syndrome and flushing may be precipitated by alcohol or coffee ingestion.

The **acromegalic patient** (*Fig. 3*) is easily recognised due to the gigantism, prominent mandible, thickened soft tissues, 'spade-like hands' and prominent supraorbital ridges. There may be visual field defects due to pressure from the pituitary tumour compressing the optic chiasma. A diabetic tendency should be borne in mind.

FACTORS RELATING TO DENTAL TREATMENT AND GA/LA/ IV SEDATION IN ENDOCRINE DISORDERS

The most common condition to consider is the management of the diabetic patient. The prevention of infections is important in the patient with diabetes as these can interfere with normal control. There is some evidence that effective periodontal care can improve metabolic control in those suffering from type 2 diabetes.[3] When providing treatment under LA alone it is important to check the patient has eaten that day, and taken their usual medication. The signs and symptoms of hypoglycaemia and hyperglycaemia are given in *Tables 4* and *5* respectively. When the diabetic regimen needs to be altered eg for GA, this is best done in conjunction with the patient's physician. The management should be matched to the severity of the diabetes, as well as to the planned surgical procedure.

For diabetes controlled by diet or oral hypoglycaemics undergoing relatively minor dental surgery under LA, the morning dose of oral hypoglycaemic should be omitted with monitoring of blood sugar levels and recommencement of oral hypoglycaemic therapy post operatively. For an IDDM patient undergoing major surgery, an IV infusion of insulin and dextrose and potassium may be used, with the infusion rate titrated against hourly blood sugar measurements. Potassium is required since insulin causes potassium to enter cells and thus the blood level must be replenished.

The use of supplemental steroids prior to dental surgery in patients at risk of an 'adrenal crisis' is a contentious issue[4,5] and is discussed in Chapter 2. After unilateral adrenalectomy for a Cushing's adenoma, steroid support may be required for a period of weeks or months and the patient's physician should be consulted. After adrenal surgery for phaeochromocytoma, steroid supplementation may rarely be required if the adrenal cortex has been damaged at operation. A GA should not be given to the uncontrolled patient with phaeochromocytoma. Local anaesthetics containing epinephrine should be avoided. Treatment may also be complicated by dysrhythmias and hypertension. Elective treatment should be carried out when the phaeochromocytoma has been treated. If emergency treatment is necessary, the blood pressure should first be controlled by the patient's physician.

A GA may precipitate a thyroid crisis in the untreated patient with hyperthyroidism resulting in risk of dysrhythmias. Such a crisis is characterised by dyspnoea, marked anxiety and tremor. Hyperthyroidism must therefore be controlled before GA is contemplated. With appropriate management, this complication should not arise in modern day practice. A treated hypothyroid patient may lapse into hyperthyroidism and this must obviously be considered if a GA is planned. Indeed the use of general anaesthesia and sedation in patients who are hypothyroid must be performed with great care and should only be carried out in specialist units. The use of local anaesthetics containing epinephrine is not contraindicated in patients receiving thyroid replacement therapy. The only time epinephrine should be avoided is during thyroid storm[6] ie extreme hyperthyroidism due to thyroid surgery, infection or trauma.

GA or IV sedation should avoided in the first trimester and last month of pregnancy. There is an increased tendency to vomiting, particularly in the last trimester due to the impaired competence of the lower oesophageal sphincter secondary mainly to pressure from the gravid uterus.

The prescription of some drugs by dentists is affected by concurrent endocrine therapy. Erythromycin may interact with diabetic medications, for example combined therapy with chlorpropamide may produce liver damage and concurrent use with glibenclamide may precipitate hypoglycaemia. There may be a reduced efficacy of oral contraceptives during therapy with antibiotics. Although the evidence for this is scarce it is wise to recommend other methods of contraception during antibiotic therapy.[7] Similarly, carbamazepine, which may be prescribed for the treatment of trigeminal neuralgia, may decrease the efficacy of the OCP and patients must be warned of this hazard.

EFFECTS OF DRUGS USED IN ENDOCRINE DISORDERS ON ORO-DENTAL STRUCTURES

The impact of corticosteroids on dental treatment was mentioned above. Other drugs used in the management of endocrine disorders may affect the mouth and surrounding structures.

Insulin given by injection may cause pain and swelling of the salivary glands. The oral hypoglycaemic metformin may produce a metallic taste.[8] Sulphonylurea hypoglycaemics such as gliclazide and glibenclamide have been implicated in causing oral lichenoid eruptions, erythema multiforme and orofacial neuropathy such as burning tongue.

Hormone replacement therapy with oestrogens may increase gingivitis and cause gingival pigmentation. The OCP may increase gingival and periodontal disease. The amount of gingival exudate is increased in women taking the OCP[9] and there is a correlation between the level of progesterone in plasma and gingival inflammation.[10]

Calcitonin may cause taste disturbance.

SUMMARY

A good basic knowledge of endocrine disorders is essential for safe dental practice. The multisystem effects of various endocrine disorders should be remembered.

1. Shafer W G, Hine M K, Levy B W. *A Textbook of Oral Pathology* 4th ed. pp 658 – 661. Philadelphia: Saunders, 1983.

2. Shlossman M, Knowler W C, Pettit D J, Genco R J. Type 2 diabetes mellitus and periodontal disease. *J Am Dent Assoc* 1990; **121:** 532- 536.

3. Simpson T C, Needleman I, Wild S H, Moles D R, Mills E J. Treatment of periodontal disease for glycaemic control in people with diabetes. Cochrane Database Syst. Rev. 2010 May 12; 5: CD004714.

4. Luyk N H, Anderson J, Ward-Booth R P. Corticosteroid therapy and the dental patient. *Br Dent J* 1985; **159:** 12 – 17.

5. Thomason J M, Girdler N M, Kendall-Taylor P, Wastell H, Weddell A, Seymour R A. An investigation into the need for supplementary steroids in organ transplant patients undergoing gingival surgery. *J Clin Periodontol* 1999; **26:** 577-582.

6. Meechan J G, Jastak J T, Donaldson D.The use of epinephrine in dentistry. *J Can Dent Assoc*; 1994; **60:** 825 - 834.

7. Hersh E V. Adverse drug interactions in dental practice: interactions involving antibiotics. *J Am Dent Assoc* 1999; **130:** 236-251.

8. Seymour R A, Meechan J G, Walton J G. *Adverse Drug Reactions in Dentistry 2nd ed*. p 137. Oxford: Oxford University Press, 1996.

9. Lindhe J, Bjorn A L. Influence of hormonal contraceptives on the gingiva of women. J *Periodont Res* 1967; **2:** 1–6.

10. Vittek J, Rappaport S C, Gordon G G, Munnangi P R, Southern A L. Concentration of circulating hormones and metabolism of androgens by human gingiva. *J Periodont* 1979; **50:** 254 – 264.

Chapter 7
Renal disorders

M. Greenwood, J. G. Meechan and D. G. Bryant*

*Consultant Oral and Maxillofacial Surgeon at Friarage Hospital, Northallerton

IN BRIEF

- Renal patients may have impaired drug excretion. Drugs used in dental sedation and general anaesthesia should be used with caution and in consultation with a physician.
- Renal disease influences the use of other drugs in dentistry, particularly NSAIDS and some antimicrobials.
- Platelet dysfunction may occur in renal patients giving rise to a bleeding tendency. Patients on haemodialysis may be heparinised. Dental treatment should be carried out on the day after dialysis. Renal condition is optimal at this time and the anticoagulant effect has stopped.
- The arm with vascular access for dialysis (the surgically created arterio-venous fistula) should not be used for venepuncture by the dentist.
- Patients who have had a kidney transplant may need corticosteroid cover, have a bleeding tendency if anticoagulated, may have gingival hyperplasia if taking ciclosporin and are prone to infection due to immunosuppression.

Patients with kidney disorders are increasingly encountered in dental practice due to improvements in medical care leading to prolonged life expectancy. In order to provide appropriate and safe dental care for these patients it is important to have a working knowledge of renal disorders and related problems.

POINTS IN THE HISTORY

The principal renal condition that the dental practitioner is likely to encounter is **chronic renal failure**. Occasionally, patients with **nephrotic syndrome** are seen (see later). It is not uncommon to encounter patients who have undergone a **renal transplant**.

It is worth bearing in mind that there is significant potential for renal problems in diabetic patients. **Diabetic nephropathy** is the most common cause of end-stage renal failure (ESRF) in developing countries and

accounts for 14% of those patients affected in the UK. It is unlikely that the dentist would be the first to diagnose diabetes mellitus, but suspicion should be raised in patients who show a changing profile of dental disease such as newly presenting or rapidly progressive periodontal disease. Further questioning may elicit that the patient feels the need to drink plenty of fluids and appears to susceptible to infections including dental abscesses and fungal conditions.[1,2]

Chronic renal failure (CRF), now often referred to as 'chronic kidney disease' (CKD), occurs after progressive kidney damage and constitutes a low glomerular filtration rate persisting over a period of three months or more. The symptoms and signs vary depending on the degree of malfunction. In early CKD the patient may notice a need to urinate frequently at night (nocturia) or may notice an uncharacteristically poor appetite. Adult CKD leads to hypertension and uraemia (a clinical and biochemical syndrome constituting end-stage renal disease). CKD can affect diverse body systems and these are summarised in *Table 1*. This can have wide ranging implications on patient management.[3]

Bone disease or '**renal osteodystrophy**' is an almost universal feature of CKD and may take one or a combination of forms. As a result of an increase in plasma phosphate levels, there is a consequent suppression of plasma calcium resulting in an elevated parathormone (PTH) level. Calcium metabolism is further compromised by disruption in vitamin D metabolism. There is a failure in conversion of 25-hydroxycholecalciferol to the active form 1, 25-dihydroxycholecalciferol. This results in secondary hyperparathyroidism. Hyperparathyroidism is discussed in more detail in Chapter 6. Many patients have been taking **steroids**, either to combat renal disease or to avoid transplant rejection. Steroids are well known to produce osteoporosis after prolonged use and this may become evident following a renal transplant.

Renal disease almost invariably causes an anaemia. This occurs mainly due to failure of production of erythropoietin (EPO) by the kidney. Renal loss of red blood cells, marrow fibrosis and increased red cell fragility with subsequent early destruction also contribute. The anaemia may result in tiredness and decreased concentration. Shortage of breath and palpitations due to decreased oxygen carriage and increased cardiac output may also occur. Marrow fibrosis leads to a reduced platelet count and poor platelet function. Patients may give a history of taking recombinant EPO, having multiple transfusions and taking iron supplements.

It is worth asking which type of dialysis a patient undergoes and when the last session was since patients are best treated when they have recently dialysed. Haemodialysis may be carried out in the body (**peritoneal**) or outside (**extra- corporeal**). Both types rely on the patient's blood being exposed to a solution hypotonic in metabolites across a semi-permeable membrane. Extra-corporeal dialysis relies upon a high flow of blood from the patient to the dialysis machine and then back to the patient. The dialysis team produce a peripheral **arterio-venous fistula** for regular large vessel diameter access (*Fig. 1*). It is of vital importance that the fistula is well-maintained and not used for any other purpose. Accidental damage to the area can result in torrential haemorrhage. Peritoneal dialysis uses the patient's own peritoneal membrane as the semi-permeable barrier. The dialysing fluid is instilled into the peritoneal cavity, left *in-situ* and drained as effluent. Infection of the peritoneal catheter is a major potential complication leading to peritonitis. Dialysis itself still carries a risk of infection (HIV, hepatitis, bacterial) and this should be borne in mind.

Haemostasis is impaired to varying degrees in patients with CKD and enquiry regarding any bleeding tendency should be made. The main factors involved are impaired platelet adhesiveness, decreased von Willebrand's factor and decreased thromboxane. Prostacyclin levels are raised leading to vasodilatation. The bleeding time is often prolonged. In addition, patients who are being dialysed will be heparinised during dialysis. However, as the effects of heparin are not prolonged treatment performed on a day when the patient is not being dialysed presents no problem with drug-induced anti-coagulation.

Infections tend to be poorly controlled in a patient with CKD and patients **post-kidney transplant** are immunosuppressed to prevent rejection. Signs of infection tend to be masked particularly in patients taking steroids and therefore care needs to be taken to treat odontogenic infections promptly and effectively. Transplant

Table 1 Clinical features of chronic renal failure (chronic kidney disease) - a systemic approach
• Cardiovascular
Hypertension
Congestive cardiac failure
Atheroma
• Gastrointestinal
Anorexia, nausea, vomiting
Peptic ulcer
• Neurological
Lassitude
Headaches
Tremor
Sensory disturbances
• Dermatological
Itching
Hyperpigmentation
• Haematological/Immunological
Bleeding tendency
Anaemia
Susceptibility to infection
• Metabolic 'Uraemia'
Thirst
Nocturia/polyuria
Electrolyte disturbances
Secondary hyperparathyroidism

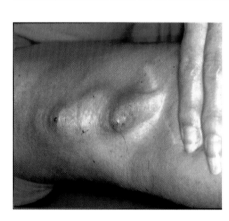

Fig. 1 A surgically created arterio-venous fistula in the antecubital fossa. A thrill is present on palpating the skin over the fistula

patients have an overall mortality of less than 5% and steroids will be used as part of the immunosuppression as well as other agents, usually **ciclosporin**. The increased risk of infection in these patients should be remembered. Patients may give a history of oral candidosis or oral viral infections eg herpes simplex, cytomegalovirus and Epstein-Barr virus (EBV). There is an increased chance of malignancy due to immunosuppression and these may range from **lymphomas** to **cutaneous cancers** eg basal cell (*Fig. 2*) and squamous cell cancers.

The **nephrotic syndrome** is found in some patients. This comprises proteinuria, hypoalbuminaemia, oedema and hyperlipidaemia. Causes include diabetes mellitus and Systemic Lupus Erythematosus. An increase in the level of circulating factor VIII leads to hypercoagulability and the possibility of thromboses. As a result such patients may give a history of taking prophylactic heparin. A patient with nephrotic syndrome may also be taking corticosteroids and using a low salt and high protein diet. . There is an increased likelihood of atheroma in these patients.

Kidney stones are of little relevance to dental practice, except for the fact that they may be associated with hyperparathyroidism. A summary of salient points to be obtained in the history is given in *Table 2*.

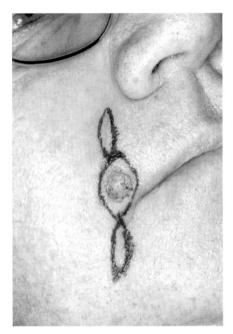

Fig. 2 A patient with a facial basal cell cancer due to immunosuppression after a kidney transplant. The patient is 'marked up' prior to surgical excision

EXAMINATION OF THE DENTAL PATIENT WITH RENAL DISEASE

Oedema may occur as a result of sodium retention and may be evident both at the ankles and around the face. **Periorbital oedema** is often seen and the patient may exhibit the characteristic 'moon face' of steroid therapy. The fluid retention may lead to pulmonary oedema, pleural and cardiac effusions which may present as shortage of breath and an inability to lie flat during dental treatment. **Bone pain** may result from a disruption of vitamin D metabolism.

The incidence of **oral ulceration** is increased in these patients and the oral mucosa may be pale secondary to anaemia but this sign is often rather subjective. As mentioned previously dental infections may become widespread very rapidly and oral candidosis may be present. Herpes simplex, zoster, cytomegalovirus, EBV and toxoplasmosis are increased in incidence and prophylactic aciclovir may be used.

Gingival hyperplasia occurs with ciclosporin therapy.[4] It is also associated with an increased and rapid build up of calculus. The hyperplasia often improves with improved oral hygiene involving scaling and polishing.

The dentist should be aware that there is an increased incidence in disorders that can be related to immunosuppression including lymphoma, skin cancers (*Fig. 2*), hairy leukoplakia, leukoplakia and Kaposi's Sarcoma.[5] Any renal transplant patient with a suspicious lesion should be referred urgently for specialist investigation. Lip cancers appear to be more likely during function of the transplanted kidney, the incidence regressing during failure of transplant and return to dialysis.[6]

Patients undergoing dialysis may experience swelling of the major salivary glands (especially the parotid glands). Salivary flow may be decreased in CKD leading to increased oral problems.[7] Palatal and buccal keratosis is sometimes seen. The conditions tend to resolve with established dialysis or transplant. The tongue may be dry and coated. Periodontal disease may be evident and there may be bleeding from the gingival margins. In children, CKD leads to decreased growth and sometimes delayed tooth eruption and enamel hypoplasia. A summary of clinical features which may be encountered in CKD is shown in *Table 1*.

The patient may have an **arteriovenous fistula** at the wrist or in the antecubital fossa (*Fig. 1*). High blood flow through the fistula leads to a palpable vibration or thrill when the examiner's fingers are placed lightly on the skin over the area of the fistula. As mentioned earlier, this arm should not be used for routine venepuncture or IV sedation.

DENTAL MANAGEMENT OF PATIENTS WITH RENAL DISORDERS (TABLE 3)

It is important to appreciate the problems faced by a patient with chronic renal disease and anticipating their reduced resistance to infection as well as their concurrent disease. Routine dental care requires little modification but it is obvious from the above that oral hygiene is important. Standard procedures should be employed to prevent cross-infection. Infiltration

Table 2 Points of relevance in the history of a patient with a renal disorder

• History of diabetes mellitus
• Chronic kidney disease (CKD)
• Related bony disorders
• Anaemia
• Dialysis - type
          - how often
          - presence of A-V fistula
• Transplant - when ?
        - associated medication including steroids
• Susceptibility to infections/recent history of repeated infection (dental or generalised)

Table 3 Management considerations in dental patients with renal disorders
• Awareness of reduced resistance to infection • Best treated under local anaesthesia • These patients may be taking (or have taken) corticosteroids • The day after dialysis is the optimum time for treatment • Electrolyte disturbances can predispose to cardiac arrhythmias • Impaired drug excretion leads to the need for care with drug prescriptions

analgesia is not contra-indicated but any bleeding tendency should be excluded prior to administering a nerve block.

Most patients are best treated under local anaesthetic due to the anaemia and potential electrolyte disturbances which would complicate GA. Corticosteroids are often prescribed for these patients and thus a steroid boost may be required for surgical procedures (see Chapter 2). These patients are often hypertensive and this should be considered prior to any form of treatment. It is important to ensure good haemostasis after oral surgical procedures because of this and the bleeding tendency. Patients are best treated the day after dialysis as platelet function will be optimal and the effect of the heparin will have worn off. Consultation with the renal physician is advised. Desmospressin (DDAVP) has been used to assist with haemostasis in cases of prolonged bleeding.

Renal disease progresses at a varying rate ranging from subclinical loss of renal reserve to renal insufficiency culminating in ESRF. Loss of reserve may not manifest itself unless the kidneys are placed under stress. This can happen after the administration of certain drugs, a heavy dietary protein load or pregnancy. Swallowed blood acts as a protein load and may occur, for example, from a post-extraction haemorrhage. Dietary manipulation is useful in decreasing sodium and potassium load and a low protein diet reduces the need to excrete nitrogenous metabolites.

The patient's cardiovascular status should be considered since these patients are predisposed to arrhythmias due to electrolyte disturbances and the incidence of atheroma is increased in patients with nephrotic syndrome, as stated earlier. Congestive cardiac failure may ensue and such patients are best treated sitting up to minimise pulmonary oedema and avoidance of placing the legs in a dependent position, again to minimise oedema.

Impaired drug excretion leads to the need for care with drug prescriptions and is discussed in the next section.

PRESCRIBING FOR PATIENTS WITH RENAL DISEASE.

Renal disease influences the use of drugs in dentistry. Many drugs prescribed by dentists are excreted by the kidney.[8] Failure to excrete a drug or its metabolites may lead to toxicity. As a general rule any drug that is nephrotoxic (such as gentamicin which used to be used in prophylaxis against endocarditis) should be avoided. Other drugs may require dose reduction. Erythromycin is contra-indicated in patients who have had a kidney transplant and are taking ciclosporin. Ciclosporin metabolism is reduced leading to an increase in toxicity.[9]

Drugs contained in the *Dental Practitioners Formulary* whose dose should be reduced in the presence of significant kidney disease include the antimicrobials aciclovir, amoxicillin, ampicillin, cefalexin and eythromicin. Tetracyclines other than doxicycline should be avoided. Non-steroidal analgesics should not be prescribed in those with more than mild renal impairment, paracetamol being the drug of choice for post-operative pain control. Drugs used in dental sedation should be used with extreme care as a greater effect than normal may be produced. The British National Formulary[10] summarises the advice concerning the prescription of drugs in patients with renal dysfunction.

CONCLUSION

Renal disease impacts on dental management. The timing of treatment may be affected in patients with serious renal impairment. Co-operation with the physician is necessary in such patients.

1. Harrison G A, Schultz T A, Schaberg S J. Deep neck infection complicated by diabetes mellitus. Report of a case. *Oral Surg Oral Med Oral Path* 1983; **55:** 133- 137.
2. Ueta E, Osaki T, Yoneda K, Yamamoto T. Prevalence of diabetes mellitus in odontogenic infections and oral candidiasis: an analysis of neutrophil suppression. *J Oral Path Oral Med* 1993; **22:** 168 – 174.
3. De Rossi S S, Glick M. Dental considerations for the patient with renal disease receiving haemodialysis. *J Am Dent Assoc* 1996; **127:** 211 – 219.
4. Seymour R A, Jacobs D J. Cyclosporin and the gingival tissues. *J Clin Perio* 1992; **19:** 1- 11.
5. Seymour R A, Thomason J M, Nolan A. Oral lesions in organ transplant patients. *J Oral Path Oral Med* 1997; **26:** 297 – 304.
6. van Leeuwen M T, Webster A C, McCredie M R, Stewart J H, McDonald S P, Amin J, Kaldor J M, Chapman J R, Vajdic C M, Grulich A E. Effect of reduced immunosuppression after kidney transplant failure on risk of cancer: population based retrospective cohort study. *Brit Med J.* 2010; 340: c570.doi:10.1136/bmj.c570
7. Kao C H, Hsieh J F, Tsai S C, Ho Y J, Chang H R. Decreased salivary function in patients with end-stage renal disease requiring haemodialysis. *Am J Kidney Diseases* 2000; **36:** 1110 – 1114.
8. Seymour R A, Meechan J G, Walton J G. *Adverse Drug Reactions in Dentistry 2nd ed.* pp 169 – 175. Oxford: Oxford University Press, 1996.
9. Jensen C W B, Flechner S M, Van Buren C T, Frazier O H, Cooley D A, Lorber M I, Kahan B D. Exacerbation of cyclosporin toxicity by concomitant administration of erythromycin. *Transplantation* 1987; **43:** 263 – 270.
10. British National Formulary. Online at http://bnf.org.

Chapter 8
The musculoskeletal system

M. Greenwood and J. G. Meechan

IN BRIEF
- Musculoskeletal disorders can affect co-operation during dental treatment
- Musculoskeletal disorders may affect oro-facial function
- Musculoskeletal disorders can affect the structure and eruption of the dentition
- Sedation with benzodiazepines is contra-indicated in some muscular diseases
- Drugs used to control musculoskeletal disease may affect oral structures

Disorders of the musculoskeletal system may impact on dental management in diverse ways. Diseases of the bones may have a direct influence on treatment and joint disorders can also cause difficulties. Cervical spine involvement may lead to poor neck extension causing difficulties in providing dental treatment under local anaesthesia or allowing the provision of a safe general anaesthetic. Muscular disorders may mitigate against safe general anaesthesia. As with all medical disorders a thorough history can help to prevent many of the possible problems which may occur secondary to musculoskeletal diseases.

POINTS IN THE HISTORY

These can be divided into diseases of bone, joint disorders and relevant soft tissue disorders. If the patient gives a history of radiotherapy to the head and neck region, the possibility of irradiation of the maxilla or mandible should be borne in mind. Dental extractions in such patients should be avoided if possible due to the risk of osteoradionecrosis (death of bone due to endarteritis obliterans).

DISORDERS OF BONE

Osteoporosis is a condition in which there is a deficiency of bone matrix and calcium salts. Bone which fractures easily is the principal complication. Patients will often complain of low back pain due to vertebral collapse. The bone is structurally normal but there is a deficiency of it. Hormone Replacement Therapy in the post-menopausal female decreases the severity of the disorder. Osteoporosis is considered a major risk factor for periodontal disease. Many patients with osteoporosis will be taking bisphosphonates. These drugs alter osteoclast function and can lead to osteonecrosis after dental extraction (see Chapter 16).

Fibrous dysplasia may affect a single bone (monostotic) or multiple bones (polyostotic). It consists of an area of bone replaced by fibrous tissue leading to local swelling. In the polyostotic disorder there may be associated skin pigmentation (café au lait patches). Rarely there may be mucosal pigmentation. The disease is usually self-limiting although in the craniofacial region it may interfere with occlusion and vision.[1] In cases of polyostotic fibrous dysplasia associated with pigmentation and precocious puberty in females the name Albright's Syndrome is applied. Radiographically the bone has a ground glass appearance. Serum calcium and phosphate levels are normal. Surgical treatment consists of 'debulking' lesions.

Paget's Disease of bone is a condition in which there is progressive bone enlargement. There is a male predominance. The prevalence of this disease appears to be decreasing.[2] The disorder consists of alternating bone deposition and resorption. Initially there may be no symptoms but later, bone pain and deformities may become evident. There is an increased likelihood of pathological fracture and there may be cranial nerve compression. The bone is hypervascular which can ultimately lead to high output cardiac failure. Rarely, an osteosarcoma may develop in Paget's Disease. Diagnosis is made by clinical and radiographic features and the blood alkaline phosphatase level is greatly increased. The skull may show a large irregular area of radiolucency-osteoporosis circumscripta and the bone is described as having a 'cotton wool' appearance. There may be hypercementosis. These patients are susceptible to chronic suppurative osteomyelitis. In view of the hypercementosis extractions will often need to be 'surgical' and carried out under antibiotic cover.

Osteopetrosis signifies a condition in which the bone density is increased but the bone is nevertheless structurally weak. The patient may suffer fractures or bone pain but is often asymptomatic. Decreased marrow activity may lead to anaemia. Some patients may be taking corticosteroids. These patients are prone to osteomyelitis or fracture. Dental extractions should be as atraumatic as possible, flaps should be avoided if possible and extractions should be carried out under antibiotic cover.

Cleidocranial dysplasia occurs as a result of a defect in membrane bone formation inherited as autosomal dominant. It involves mainly the skull and clavicles. The head is large and brachycephalic with a persistent frontal suture. The clavicles are absent or stunted conferring the ability to approximate the shoulders anteriorly (*Fig. 1*). There is a persistent deciduous dentition, often unerupted permanent teeth, dentigerous cysts and supernumeraries.[3]

Osteogenesis imperfecta is a rare autosomal dominant condition consisting of a defect in collagen formation. It may be associated with dentinogenesis imperfecta. The patient may give a history of multiple fractures secondary to relatively minor trauma. There may be associated deafness and the patients tend to have weak tendons and bruise easily. Heart valve problems may occur. It is rare to fracture the jaw as a result of dental treatment.

Rickets and **osteomalacia** may occur in conditions of defective skeletal mineralisation, the former occurring in children ('knock knees') and the latter in adults. The conditions are usually related to a deficiency of intake or absorption of vitamin D. Osteomalacia is sometimes seen in patients with chronic kidney disease. Excess osteoid matrix at the costochondral rib junction leads to the appearance of a so-called 'Rickety Rosary'. Dental defects are seen only in severe cases. When there is associated malabsorption the possibility of reduced vitamin K uptake should be considered, as this may affect blood clotting.

A patient with **achondroplasia** would be obvious as the classic 'circus dwarf'. The condition arises due to a defect in cartilaginous bone formation and is inherited as autosomal dominant. The relevance to dentistry

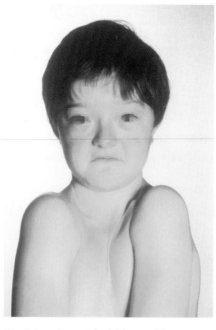

Fig. 1 A patient with cleidocranial dysplasia. The clavicles are absent or stunted due to a defect in membrane bone formation

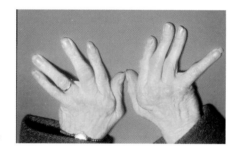

Fig. 2 The fingers are deviated to the ulnar side in this patient with rheumatoid arthritis

is that the incidence of malocclusion is increased and patients may have a diabetic tendency.

JOINT DISEASE

Osteoarthritis may occur as a 'wear and tear' phenomenon and occurs due to a degeneration of articular cartilage. It has characteristic radiographic appearances (see later). There are no systemic symptoms. Treatment is mainly by reduction in weight if required when the disease affects weight bearing joints, physiotherapy, local application of heat and anti-inflammatories which may lead to a bleeding tendency.

Rheumatoid arthritis is a multisystem disorder which is thought to be autoimmune in nature. One theory

Table 1 The multisystem nature of rheumatoid arthritis

- Cardiovascular - Myocarditis
  - Pericarditis
  - Valve inflammation
- Respiratory - Pulmonary nodules/ fibrosis
- Renal - Amyloidosis
- Liver - Hepatic impairment
- Skin - Palmar erythema
  - Subcutaneous 'rheumaoid nodules
- General - Malaise
  - Anaemia of chronic disease
  - Thrombocytopaenia

is that an autoantibody to abnormal immunoglobulin in joint tissues leads to the formation of an antigen-antibody complex which activates complement causing inflammation and synovial damage. The mean age of onset is between 30 and 40 years, the juvenile form is known as Still's Disease. There is a female predominance.

Juvenile chronic arthritis may lead to an increased incidence of caries and periodontal disease.[4] In addition, if the TMJ is involved facial growth may be disturbed,[5] however, the condylar condition can improve with age.[6] One of the early signs of development of rheumatoid arthritis may be stiffness of the fingers, particularly in the early morning ('early morning stiffness') which usually decreases during the day. In more advanced disease the direction of the fingers appear to drift away from the thumb (ulnar deviation) (*Fig. 2*). The onset is often slow but it can be acute with malaise, fever and joint pain. There is anaemia which is normocytic and normochromic - the so-called anaemia of chronic disease. Treatment in the early stages is usually with nonsteroidal anti-inflammatory drugs. Second line treatment includes a variety of agents such as gold and the chemotherapy agent methotrexate (this may lead to folic acid deficiency with the potential for secondary oral problems). Corticosteroids have been used for treatment as have antimalarial medications. The mainstay of physical treatment involves occupational therapy and includes household

THE MUSCULOSKELETAL SYSTEM

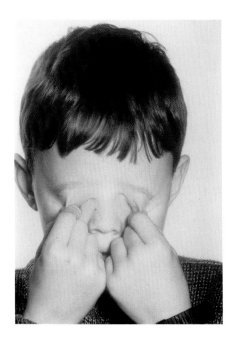

Fig. 3 Hyperelasticity of the skin in a patient with Ehler's-Danlos Syndrome

device modification eg modified toothbrush handles, modified kitchen appliances. *Table 1* lists the potential multisystem manifestations of rheumatoid arthritis. The recommendation of electric toothbrushes for these and other patients with musculoskeletal disorders should be considered to aid oral hygiene. **Felty's Syndrome** consists of rheumatoid arthritis, splenomegaly leading to leucopaenia, anaemia and lymphadenopathy.

The skin disorder psoriasis may have an associated arthritis which usually resembles a less severe version of a rheumatoid arthritis. Blood tests are normal, oral lesions are rare. Occasionally treatment might be with methotrexate.

Gout may be of primary or secondary type. In primary gout there are raised serum levels of uric acid leading to the deposition of urates especially in joints leading to arthritis. In secondary gout certain drug treatments may precipitate the condition. An alcoholic binge can instigate gout in those predisposed to it. Gouty tophi may occur where masses of urate crystals become deposited in joints or extra-articular sites eg the subcutaneous nodules of the helix of the ear. The classic joint affected by gout is that of the great toe. Gout may lead to renal failure. The treatment in an

acute attack is usually indomethacin but longer term maintenance requires allopurinol which decreases uric acid production.

In patients with prosthetic **joint replacements** there is no indication for antibiotic cover for dental treatment[7,8] but there is a suggestion of a degree of immunocompromise in rheumatoid arthritis and thus antibiotic cover may be wise for these patients. The same may be said of the patient with diabetes mellitus who has a prosthetic joint.

OTHER DISORDERS

Ankylosing spondylitis is a chronic inflammatory disease mainly of young males, affecting the spine. Over 90% of cases are HLA B27 positive - the disease is partly genetically determined. There is ossification of ligaments and tendons and the onset is insidious. The patient often complains of low back pain. A quarter of patients may develop eye lesions. Patients may also have aortic valvular disease or cardiac conduction defects. As intervertebral ossification develops the radiograph takes on a so-called 'bamboo spine' appearance. Treatment is with anti-inflammatory medications. There are implications for general anaesthesia and these are discussed later. **Reiter's Disease** consists of the triad of arthritis, urethritis and conjunctivitis. Like patients with ankylosing spondylitis a majority of patients are HLA B27 positive. They are usually 20 to 40-year-old males.

Marfan's Syndrome is an autosomal dominant condition which comprises skeletal, ocular and cardiovascular malformations. The patients are conspicuously tall and have lax ligaments. They have a predisposition to lung cysts leading to risk of pneumothorax. Ocular lens dislocation can occur. Aortic dissection is a possibility leading to aortic and mitral valve incompetence. The palatal vault is high and there is an increased incidence of TMJ dysfunction. There may be associated cardiac disease.

In **Ehlers-Danlos syndrome** the patient's principal complaints are of lax joints and bruising easily (there

Table 2 Points in the history which may be of relevance in musculoskeletal disease
• **Bone Disorders** Osteoporosis Rickets and osteomalacia Fibrous dysplasia Paget's disease of bone Osteopetrosis Cleidocranial dysostosis Osteogenesis imperfecta Achondroplasia
• **Joint Disorders** Osteoarthritis Rheumatoid arthritis Psoriatic arthritis Gout Mouth opening Neck extension
• **Other Disorders** Ankylosing spondylitis Marfan's syndrome Ehler's-Danlos syndrome Reiter's syndrome
• **Muscular Disorders** Duchenne muscular dystrophy Polymyositis Dermatomyositis Cranial arteritis Polymyalgia rheumatica

may be deficient platelet function). The skin is elastic (*Fig. 3*) and there is a predisposition to mitral valve prolapse. This disorder of collagen formation (of which there are various sub-types) may be autosomal dominant but some types are recessive.

Myasthenia gravis is an autoimmune disease of the neuromuscular junction involving the post junctional acetylcholine receptors. The condition is characterised by muscle weakness. Ocular, facial and pharyngeal muscles may be involved. The condition is described in more detail in Chapter 4.

Muscular disorders may be of relevance in dental treatment. **Duchenne muscular dystrophy is** a sex-linked disorder comprising widespread muscle weakness which tends not to affect the head and neck but may be relevant in terms of ease of access to treatment or provision of general anaesthesia or sedation (see later). The affected muscles appear to be enlarged - pseudohypertrophy. Cardiomyopathy and respiratory impairment may occur. Acquired myopathies include **polymyositis** and **dermatomyositis** (the latter if there is an associated skin disorder). These are rare and immunologically mediated inflammatory myopathies comprising pain and muscle weakness. There are often circulating autoantibodies present. The female incidence is twice that of the male. Speech and swallowing may be difficult. The characteristic rash may occur in up to a third of cases of polymyositis which consists of a butterfly-shaped violet rash across the bridge of the nose and cheeks. There may be associated Raynaud's Disease (a vasospastic disorder resulting in excessive reaction of extremities to cold) or other connective tissue disorders eg Sjögren's Syndrome. Treatment often involves corticosteroids.

Cranial arteritis and **polymyalgia rheumatica** (PMR) are disorders of blood vessels but cause muscle pain due to ischaemia. Inflammation with luminal obliteration of the medium sized arteries occurs. Giant cells may be found histologically thus the arteritis is a giant cell type. The affected area may be cranial/temporal or more widespread in the case of PMR. In cranial arteritis the eye can be involved leading to blindness. In this form of arteritis there is a unilateral throbbing headache usually affecting middle aged or older females. A biopsy of the temporal artery confirms the diagnosis. Early administration of prednisolone is mandatory if the disorder is suspected to prevent blindness. Ischaemic pain may be felt in the muscles of mastication and this must be differentiated from TMJ pain. Unlike TMJ pain it tends to have a later onset ie middle aged or older and there is no diurnal variation. The pain is more severe and there is an increased erythrocyte sedimentation rate (ESR). In trigeminal neuralgia the pain may be associated with mastication but the ESR is normal and it may thus be differentiated from cranial arteritis. In cases of PMR a similar age and sex distribution is seen compared to cranial arteritis.

A summary of salient points to be obtained in the history is given in *Table 2*.

Table 3 Summary of points on examination of a dental patient with a musculoskeletal disorder		
• Joint Disorders	-	Gait
	-	Swelling, deformity
	-	Heberden's nodes (see text)
	-	Rheumatoid hands
	-	Subcutaneous nodules in rheumatoid arthritis
• Osteogenesis imperfecta	-	Blue sclera, may be brown heavily worn teeth if dentinogenesis imperfecta associated
• Cleidocranial dysplasia	-	Large, brachycephalic head
	-	Hypoplastic maxilla
	-	Absent/hypoplastic clavicles
• Marfan's Syndrome	-	Tall stature
	-	Long fingers
	-	High arched palate
	-	Lax ligaments
• Osteoporosis	-	Vertebral collapse possibly leading to spinal deformity
• Fibrous Dysplasia	-	Localised areas of 'swelling' of skeleton(may be associated with skin pigmentation)
• Paget's disease of bone	-	Sabre tibia
	-	Increased head circumference
	-	Increased alveolar ridge width
• Ankylosing spondylitis	-	Flexed/hunched appearance to back
• Muscle disorders	-	May be altered speech/muscle tone
• Dermatomyositis	-	Violet/purple butterfly rash over bridge of nose/cheek
• Cranial arteritis	-	Tender, prominent temporal artery

EXAMINATION

The dental patient may have signs which can be related to their musculoskeletal disorder. A summary is given in *Table 3*. The patient with osteogenesis imperfecta may have the classic blue sclera, for example (*Fig. 4*). If there is associated dentinogenesis imperfecta, the teeth may have a brown discolouration with marked attrition due to the weakened tooth substance.

Joint disorders may be suspected from the patient's gait or a deformity may be evident. The osteoarthritic patient may have nodules close to the distal interphalangeal joints of the fingers - so-called Heberden's Nodes. The radiographic appearances of osteoarthritis are characteristic with reduced joint space, subchondral bone cysts and sclerosis and lipping of osteophytes at the joint margins. TMJ function does not appear to be correlated with the radiographic appearance. Patients with rheumatoid arthritis may complain of systemic symptoms in addition to those of the joints. The fingers may be deviated to the ulnar side ie away from the thumb. There may be redness over the small joints of the hands and feet and palmar erythema. Rheumatoid nodules are sometimes seen - the principal site being near the elbow on the extensor surface of the arm. Radiographic examination shows a widened joint space and the shadows of associated soft tissue swelling. The adjacent bone may be osteoporotic. Sjögren's syndrome may be associated. Radiographic changes are common in the TMJ and include erosions and flattening of the condylar head. As with osteoarthritis, major TMJ problems are not necessarily associated. Still's disease may be complicated by bony ankylosis.

The oral complications of radiotherapy to the oral cavity/salivary glands are summarised in *Table 4*. The most common complication is a mucositis. When osteoradionecrosis occurs the mandibular bone becomes avascular and necrotic. Overlying mucosa and skin may be destroyed and the bone exposed. An ill-fitting denture can induce a post-irradiation osteomyelitis due to mucosal ulceration.

Infective arthropathy of the TMJ is an unusual event and usually follows a penetrating injury. *Haemophilus, Staphylococcus aureus* or *Mycobacterium tuberculosis* are the common infecting organisms.

The patient with Cleidocranial dysplasia has a large, brachycephalic head with bulging frontal, parietal and occipital regions. There is a persistent metopic (frontal) suture visible radiographically and the middle third of the face is hypoplastic. The clavicles are either hypoplastic or absent leading to an ability to approximate the shoulders anteriorly.

A Marfan's patient is often suspected not only due to the tall stature, but also the long fingers and ligament laxity. Such laxity also exists in the patient with Ehler's-Danlos syndrome but here the skin is also elastic. These patients have a predisposition to bruising and a haematological cause should also be considered.

The sequelae of osteoporosis may be seen as a collapse of the spine leading to a subsequent chest deformity. There also may be decreased alveolar height due to bone loss.

The patient with fibrous dysplasia may have bilateral lesions of the maxilla giving the appearance which has been labelled 'cherubism'. The eyes are classically described as being 'upturned toward heaven'. Hyperpigmentation may be associated with the polyostotic type as mentioned earlier, the lesions are usually on the same side as the bone lesions. Radiographic examination shows a ground glass appearance of the bone.

Paget's disease of bone may be recognised by a characteristic appearance of the lower leg (being convex forward) the so-called 'sabre-tibia'. The patient may be deaf or have impaired vision secondary to cranial nerve compression. Radiographs may show a mixture of sclerosis and radiolucency giving a so-called 'cotton wool' appearance to the bone (*Fig. 5*). Symmetrical malar bulging may occur giving the appearance

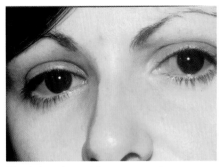

Fig. 4 A patient with osteogenesis imperfecta with the classic blue sclera

of so-called 'leontiasis ossea'. The alveolar ridges may be widened and radiographic examination of the teeth may reveal a loss of lamina dura as well as hypercementosis.

Ankylosing spondylitis may be recognised by the flexed or hunched appearance of the back. On radiographic examination the spine has a 'bamboo' appearance. There may be restricted mouth opening.

The patient with Reiter's syndrome has an arthritis, urethritis and conjunctivitis. There is an associated keratotic thickening of the skin of the soles of hands and feet - a condition known as keratoderma blenorrhagica. Oral lesions include white patches with a surrounding red area which are painless, transient and may affect any part of the mouth.

Muscular disorders may be suspected from the patient's gait or their speech. A waddling gait develops in Duchenne muscular dystrophy along with the pseudohypertrophy of muscles mentioned earlier. In the facioscapulohumeral type there is a lack of facial expression. The myotonic disorders are characterised by slow muscle relaxation after contraction. If the tongue is affected dysarthria results. Ptosis may be evident and there is atrophy of the muscles of mastication. Intellectual deterioration also occurs.

Patients with polymyositis and dermatomyositis may have difficulties in speaking and swallowing due mainly to muscle contracture. A violet/purple butterfly-shaped facial rash may occur extending over the bridge of the nose and cheeks. There may be associated Sjögren's Syndrome. The

mouth may have a purple erythematous appearance with areas of superficial ulceration.

The patient with cranial arteritis will have little to see on clinical examination but may have a prominent temporal artery on the same side as the pain which is tender to palpation. Diagnosis is confirmed by temporal artery biopsy. Patients with PMR predominantly have painful, weak and stiff shoulders.

GENERAL AND LOCAL ANAESTHESIA, SEDATION AND MANAGEMENT CONSIDERATIONS IN THE DENTAL PATIENT WITH MUSCULOSKELETAL DISEASE

The patient with osteogenesis imperfecta may have secondary chest deformities which may be severe enough to compromise respiratory function. This should be borne in mind when assessing a patient for GA and in extreme cases, intravenous sedation. The patient with osteopetrosis may be anaemic or may be on corticosteroid therapy and both of these will have a bearing on their management. Patients with osteoporosis may have impaired respiratory function due to vertebral collapse unfavourably altering the dimensions of the thorax. In cases of fibrous dysplasia, patients are at increased risk of being hyperthyroid or having a diabetic tendency. In cases of Paget's disease of bone there is the possibility of cardiac failure and chest deformities.

The best management of osteoradionecrosis or osteonecrosis is prevention. It is sensible to complete any dental treatment prior to radiotherapy or commencement of bisphosphonate therapy. Osteoradionecrosis may follow at any time after radiotherapy but a third of cases develop in the first six months and it is particularly important to avoid extractions in the first six months to one year. In the case of pre-radiotherapy extractions, particular care should be taken to ensure that bone is covered by mucosa. Post-radiotherapy extractions should be avoided if possible but if unavoidable trauma should be kept to a minimum. Local anaesthetic without

Table 4 Potential oral complications of radiotherapy to the head and neck region.

- Osteoradionecrosis, irradiation induced osteomyelitis
- Xerostomia
- Radiation caries
- Mucositis, ulceration
- Trismus
- Candidosis
- Periodontal disease
- Taste loss

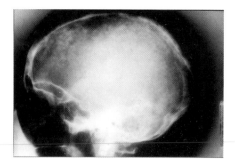

Fig 5 This 'cotton wool' appearance to the skull is seen in Paget's disease of bone.

vasoconstrictor should be used and raising of periosteum should be minimised. Any sharp bone edges should be gently trimmed. Soft tissue should be closed accurately and prophylactic antibiotics continued for at least one month. Radiation caries should be controlled by optimising oral hygiene and daily topical fluoride application may also be used.

Extracting teeth can lead to necrosis of the bone following radiotherapy to the mandible. Extractions are best avoided in the first year after radiotherapy. A preventative protocol is important. Similar considerations apply in patients taking bisphosphonates who require dental extractions.

SYNDROMIC PATIENTS

A patient with Marfan's Syndrome may have lung cysts which predispose to spontaneous pneumothorax. Curvature of the spine in an antero-posterior direction (kyphosis) and lateral direction (scoliosis) may lead to a significant diminution in respiratory function. The aortic and mitral valve incompetence may lead to cardiac symptoms. Patients with Ehler's-Danlos Syndrome are predisposed to mitral valve prolapse and conduction defects. Patients with ankylosing spondylitis may have decreased mouth opening making intubation difficult as well as causing problems with the treatment itself. Spinal deformity may lead to secondary thoracic deformity and consequent respiratory impairment. These patients may have associated aortic valvular problems.

JOINT DISORDERS

In both osteoarthritis and rheumatoid arthritis, cervical spine mobility may cause problems in positioning the patient appropriately, both in terms of facilitating treatment provision and anaesthesia. Patients with rheumatoid arthritis will frequently wear a cervical collar. Corticosteroids may be used in both types of arthritis and will often be given by local joint injection and therefore not produce a need for steroid cover. Systemic treatments may be used in some cases, however. The variety of chronic diseases associated with rheumatoid arthritis may be of relevance (*Table 1*). The TMJ in rheumatoid arthritis often does not produce pain, but there may be decreased movement ie diminished mouth opening.

Patients with gout are at increased risk of hypertension, ischaemic heart disease, diabetes mellitus and renal disease.

Other disorders

In muscular dystrophy patients, cardiomyopathy and respiratory disease should be considered. These patients are also sensitive to the muscle relaxant suxamethonium and are predisposed to developing malignant hyperthermia if a GA is used. Steroid therapy may be of significance when treating patients with cranial arteritis or PMR.

The use of benzodiazepine sedation is contra-indicated in patients with myasthenia gravis due to the muscle relaxant properties of this group of drugs.

EFFECTS OF DRUGS USED TO TREAT MUSCULOSKELETAL DISORDERS ON ORO-DENTAL STRUCTURES

The effects of corticosteroids have been discussed in Chapter 2.

Non-steroidal anti-inflammatory drugs (NSAIDs) may offer some protection against periodontal disease as they interfere with prostaglandin synthesis. COX 2 inhibitors such as celecoxib may cause stomatitis and taste disturbance.

Penicillamine may also cause taste disturbance. This latter drug has been implicated in producing lichenoid reactions and oral ulceration. In addition as it may produce a thrombocytopaenia spontaneous gingival bleeding may result.

Ciclosporin is occasionally used in the management of rheumatoid arthritis and this may cause gingival overgrowth in about 30% of patients.[9]

Methotrexate is sometimes used to treat rheumatoid arthritis and may be the cause of oral ulceration. The important point to note about methotrexate is that its toxicity is greatly increased by combined therapy with NSAIDs, corticosteroids and penicillins (including amoxicillin).[10] Combined therapy with these drugs must be avoided as fatalities may occur.

The cytokine-inhibitor agents eg adalimumab, etenarcept and infliximab, are increasingly used as second-line treatments in rheumatoid arthritis (and sometimes in ankylosing spondylitis). As a consequence of the effect of these agents on the immune response, it is important that patients are rendered dentally fit prior to the commencement of therapy. Any problems that do occur after such treatment has been started, should be treated promptly and aggressively.

Allopurinol, which is used in the management of gout may cause taste disturbance and oral paraesthesias. In addition it can produce erythema multiforme.

Sulfasalazine, which may be used in the management of rheumatoid arthritis, can cause oral ulceration, stomatitis, glossitis, lichen planus and lupus erythematosus. It may also cause parotitis. Anaemia, leucopaenia and thrombocytopaenia are other unwanted effects of this drug that can impact on surgical dentistry.

Baclofen, which is a skeletal muscle relaxant may produce xerostomia.

SUMMARY

Musculoskeletal disorders may alter the management of dental patients in diverse ways. Management may need to be altered because of medication used to combat the disorder eg steroid therapy, the nature of the disorder itself or related conditions eg pulmonary fibrosis as part of the multisystem disorder rheumatoid arthritis. As with many disorders, a thorough history will lead to safe and effective patient management.

1. Michael C B, Lee A G, Patrinely J R, Stal S, Blacklock J B. Visual loss associated with fibrous dysplasia of the anterior skull base. Case report and review of the literature. *J Neurology* 2000; **92:** 350 – 354.

2. Noor M, Shobak D. Paget's disease of bone: diagnosis and treatment update. *Curr Rheum Reps* 2000, **2:** 67 – 73.

3. Butterworth C. Cleidocranial dysplasia: modern concepts of treatment and a report of an orthodontic resistant case requiring a restorative solution. *Dent Update* 1999, **26:** 458 – 462.

4. Drecka-Kuzan K. Comparative study on the incidence of dental caries in children with rheumatoid fever and rheumatoid arthritis. *Rheumatoligial* 1971; **9:** 125-133.

5. Walton A G, Welbury R R, Foster H E, Thomason J M. Juvenile chronic arthritis: a dental review. *Oral Diseases* 1999; **5:** 68-75.

6. Twilt M, Schulten A J, Prahl-Andersen B, van Suijlekom-Smit L W. Long-term follow-up of craniofacial alterations in juvenile idiopathic arthritis. *Angle Orthod.* 2009; **79:** 1057-1062.

7. McGowan D A, Hendrey M L. Is antibiotic prophylaxis required for dental patients with joint replacements? *Br Dent J* 1985; **158:** 336 – 338.

8. Simmons N A, Ball A P, Cawson R A, Eykyn S J, Hughes S P F, McGowan D A, Shanson D C. Case against antibiotic prophylaxis for dental treatment of patients with joint prostheses. *Lancet* 1992; **339:** 301.

9. Seymour R A, Smith D G, Rogers S R. The comparative effects of azothiaprine and cyclosporin on some gingival health parameters of renal transplant patients. *J Clin Perio* 1987; **14:** 610 – 613.

10. Mayal B, Poggi G, Parkin J D. Neutropenia due to methotrexate therapy for psoriasis and rheumatoid arthritis may be fatal. *Med J Aust* 1991; **155:** 480-484.

Chapter 9
Haematology and patients with bleeding problems

M. Greenwood and J. G. Meechan

IN BRIEF

- Disorders of the blood can affect the timing of dental treatment
- White cell defects influence healing after surgical treatments
- Red cell defects influence healing and the choice of anaesthesia
- Clotting problems impact on surgical treatments and the choice of local anaesthesia
- Anti-coagulant medication interacts with drugs used in dentistry

Disorders of the blood can affect the management of dental patients. Particular oral signs may be produced. In addition, healing may be affected and the choice of anaesthesia for operative procedures will be influenced. Similarly, patients who have problems with haemostasis are a concern. Surgical procedures are obvious problems. However, restorative dentistry is not trouble-free as patients with bleeding problems may present difficulties regarding the choice of local anaesthesia, as regional block techniques may be contra-indicated in some patients.

Disorders of the blood can be categorised as

- Problems with red blood cells
- Problems with white blood cells.
   Bleeding disorders may be congenital or acquired, for example due to drug therapy. They may be due to:
- Problems with platelets
- Deficiencies in clotting factors
- Vascular problems
- Fibrinolytic problems.

POINTS IN THE HISTORY

The routine medical history taken from each patient before treatment should include enquiries about the blood and bleeding. Feelings such as lethargy may be produced by many disorders but may indicate an underlying anaemia. Repeated infections may be the result of deficiencies in white cell numbers or function. Regular nose bleeds or bruising after minor trauma should be taken seriously as should episodes of prolonged bleeding after dental extractions. Nevertheless, it is possible that a dental surgical procedure could be the first discovery of a bleeding problem in a patient otherwise thought to be normal. The authors have been involved in a case of a patient in his twenties who had undergone orthopaedic surgery uneventfully but who suffered a life-threatening bleed following the removal of third molar teeth. Investigations performed after that event provided a diagnosis of von Willebrand's disease.

A full drug history should be elicited. This is important because, in addition to detecting drugs taken to directly interfere with bleeding, such as warfarin, many drugs can produce bleeding disorders as an unwanted side effect. It is not only prescribed medication that may interfere with haemostasis; drugs of abuse including alcohol and heroin may cause excess bleeding. Finally, any family history of problems with bleeding should be elicited.

When a haematological or bleeding disorder is suspected special investigations to be performed include a full blood count and clotting studies. The ranges of normal haematological values are given in *Tables 1* and *2*.

PROBLEMS WITH RED BLOOD CELLS

Two categories of disorder may occur: these are
- Anaemia
- Polycythaemia.

Anaemia

Anaemia is a reduction in the oxygen carrying capacity of the blood. Anaemia may be caused by a number of disease states or because of drug therapy.[1] This may be the result of reduced numbers of erythrocytes or defects in haemoglobin function. Red cell numbers can be low because of decreased production due to a deficiency state or bone marrow aplasia. Alternatively, the erythrocyte numbers may be reduced because of increased destruction; this is known as haemolytic anaemia.

Deficiency anaemia can be caused by lack of iron, vitamin B_{12} or folate. The different deficiencies produce different effects on the erythrocyte. Iron deficiency produces small cells, lack of vitamin B_{12} or folate results in large erythrocytes. Deficiency states are corrected by replacement therapy. Iron deficiency may be due to dietary factors or due to loss of blood, for example from an intestinal malignancy. Vitamin B_{12} deficiency, known as pernicious anaemia, is not due to dietary problems but is caused by poor absorption of the vitamin. This is a result of defective intrinsic factor function caused by autoantibody attack. Pernicious anaemia is of interest to dentists as it is one of the complications of nitrous oxide abuse.

Haemolytic anaemia can be the result of extrinsic factors (such as malaria) or problems with haemoglobin. Included among the conditions that produce defects in haemoglobin are sickle cell disease, the thalassaemias and glucose 6-phosphate dehydrogenase deficiency. Sickle cell disease represents a variant in haemoglobin that is known as haemoglobin S. This haemoglobin causes distortion of the erythrocyte when the oxygen tension is reduced leading to increased haemolysis. Sickle cell disease is a homozygous condition. More common is the heterozygous state - sickle cell trait. This trait is normally asymptomatic and only causes problems when the patient is in a situation of reduced oxygen concentration. Sickle cell disease and trait are more common in patients of African and Afro-Caribbean descent than in other populations.

The thalassaemias may be found in patients of Asian, Mediterranean and Middle-East descent. Like sickle cell disease these conditions increase haemolysis. They are often associated with a cardiomyopathy. The thalassaemias can produce bone-marrow expansion, which can present as maxillary enlargement.

Glucose 6-phosphate dehydrogenase deficiency causes a metabolic disturbance in the erythrocyte leading to an accumulation of oxidants. These oxidants produce methaemoglobin and cause denaturing of haemoglobin with resultant haemolysis.

These can be divided into diseases of bone, joint disorders and relevant soft tissue disorders. If the patient gives a history of radiotherapy to the head and neck region, the possibility of irradiation of the maxilla or mandible should be borne in mind. Dental extractions in such patients should be avoided if possible due to the risk of osteoradionecrosis (death of bone due to irradiation obliterans).

Table 1 Normal ranges for haematological measurements in males and females.

Parameter	Normal range (male)	Normal range (female)
Red cell count	$4.5-6.5 \times 10^{12}$/L	$3.9-5.6 \times 10^{12}$/L
White cell count	$4.0 - 11.0 \times 10^9$/L	$4.0 - 11.0 \times 10^9$/L
Platelets	$50.0 - 400.0 \times 10^9$/L	$150.0 - 400.0 \times 10^9$/L
Reticulocytes	$25 - 100 \times 10^9$/L	$25 - 100 \times 10^9$/L
Erythrocyte sedimentation rate	Upper limit = (age in years ÷ 2	Upper limit = (age in years +10) ÷ 2
Haematocrit	0.4 - 0.54	0.37 - 0.47
Haemoglobin	13.5 - 18.0g/dL	11.5 - 16.0g/dL
Mean cell volume	76 - 96fl	76 - 96fl
Mean cell haemoglobin	27 - 32pg	27 - 32pg
Mean cell haemoglobin concentration	30 - 36g/dL	30 - 36g/dL
Red cell folate	$0.36 - 1.44\mu$ mol/L	$0.36 - 1.44\mu$ mol/L
Vitamin B12	0.13 - 0.68 nmol/L	0.13 - 0.68 nmol/L
Prothrombin time	10 - 14 seconds	10 - 14 seconds
Activated partial prothrombin time	35 - 45 seconds	35 - 45 seconds

Polycythaemia

Polycythaemia is the over-production of red blood cells. It may be a sign of cardiac problems that decrease the amount of blood passing through the lungs, for example a cardiac shunt from the right to the left side of the heart. A serious complication of polycythaemia is thrombosis. The condition may be controlled by frequent bloodletting or by cytotoxic drug therapy.

PROBLEMS WITH WHITE CELLS

White cell problems can present as:
- Reduced numbers (leucopaenia)
- Increased numbers (leucocytosis)
- Malignancy.

Leucopaenia

Leucopaenia is a white blood cell count of less than 4.0×10^9/L. It may be the result of a disease process such as HIV infection or the early stages of leukaemia. Alternatively it may be caused by drug therapy.[1] Cyclic neutropenia is a condition in which there are cycles where the white cell count drops. The clinical presentation of leucopaenia is known as agranulocytosis. This produces susceptibility to infection. The dentist may be involved as oral ulceration may occur with this condition.

Leucocytosis

Leucocytosis is a white cell count of greater than 11×10^9/L. Many infections raise the white cell count and it is a feature of leukaemia.

Malignancy

Malignant diseases of the white cells include:
• Leukaemias
• Lymphomas
• Myeloma.

Leukaemias

Leukaemias divided into acute and chronic forms. Two types of acute and two kinds of chronic leukaemia are recognised. These are:
• Acute lymphoblastic leukaemia (ALL)
• Acute myeloblastic leukaemia (AML)
• Chronic lymphocytic leukaemia (CLL)
• Chronic myeloid leukaemia (CML).

Acute lymphoblastic leukaemia (ALL) is the commonest presentation in children. The prognosis in children with ALL is better than that for adults for whom the long-term survival is low.

Acute myeloblastic leukaemia is more common in adults compared to children. The prognosis for both adults and children is poor.

The treatment for the acute leukaemias is with cytotoxic drug therapy or bone marrow transplantation.

The chronic leukaemias involve the proliferation of more mature cells than those found in the acute conditions. The prognosis is better than for the acute leukaemias and adults are more commonly affected than children. Chronic lymphocytic leukaemia (CLL) is the more common form. Some patients with this condition are asymptomatic. The disease may present with splenomegaly (an enlarged spleen) and lymph node enlargement. Chronic myeloid leukaemia (CML) affects adults of a slightly younger age group than CLL. Splenomegaly occurs but lymph node enlargement is not as common as with CLL. Treatment is with chemotherapy and radiotherapy.

Lymphomas

Lymphomas are divided into two types:
• Hodgkin's

• Non-Hodgkin's.

Hodgkin's lymphoma mainly affects males with the peak incidence in the fourth decade of life. It presents as lymph node enlargement. This enlargement often occurs in the neck. Non-Hodgkin's lymphomas have a poorer prognosis than the Hodgkin's type. Whereas Hodgkin's can be centred on one node Non-Hodgkin's is usually multi-focal. Burkitt's lymphoma is a condition associated with the Epstein-Barr virus and may present in the jaws. Treatment for the lymphomas is with combined chemotherapy and radiotherapy.

Myeloma

Multiple myeloma is a malignancy of plasma cells. It may present in the jaws as a radiolucency associated with loosening of the teeth and altered sensation. Treatment is with chemotherapy. Occasionally an isolated lesion (a plasmacytoma) may occur in the jaws (*Fig. 1*); these are treated by radiotherapy.

PROBLEMS WITH PLATELETS

Platelet problems may be:
• Congenital
• Acquired.

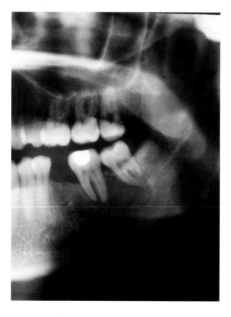

Fig. 1 A plasmacytoma presenting as a mandibular radiolucency at the lower molar apices

Table 2 Differential white cell count (normal range)	
Cell	%
Neutrophils	40-75
Eosinophils	1-6
Basophils	0-1
Lymphocytes	20-45
Monocytes	2-10

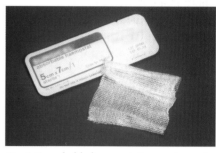

Fig. 2 Resorbable haemostatic agents can be placed in sockets to aid healing.

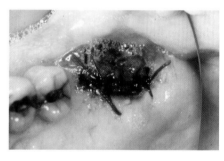

Fig. 3 A haemostatic pack held in place with sutures (courtesy Dr U.J. Moore)

The problem may be due to decreased platelet numbers or deficiencies in function. The normal platelet count is over 150 x 10⁹/L. The lowest level acceptable for dental surgery is 50 x 10⁹/L. Patients with counts of less than 100 x 10⁹/L may show prolonged bleeding but normally local measures such as suturing and the placing of a haemostatic pack can control this (*Figs 2* and *3*). Replacement therapy is required if the platelet level is less than 50 x 10⁹/L. Normally a platelet transfusion will be performed 30 minutes before surgery. If the problem is one of idiopathic thrombocytopaenia oral systemic steroids can be prescribed for 7 to 10 days pre-operatively. This can increase the platelet numbers to a suitable level.

Platelet function can be affected by disease or by drugs. Glanzmann's syndrome is a defect in platelet aggregation. A platelet infusion must be given prior to surgery as bleeding can be severe. A number of drugs interfere with platelet function. Those specifically used for this purpose include aspirin and dipyridamole. There is normally no treatment other than local measures required to obtain haemostasis in patients taking these drugs. If there is a concern in a patient taking aspirin then the drug must be stopped for at least 10 days prior to surgery as irreversible changes are produced and replacement with unaffected platelets is needed. Normally, aspirin does not produce problems.

DEFICIENCIES IN CLOTTING FACTORS

The classic example of a clotting factor deficiency is haemophilia. Haemophilia A is a sex-linked condition that varies in severity. It is due to a deficiency in Factor VIII. Factor VIII function of 25% or above of normal usually provides satisfactory clotting. Patients with levels of less than 5% will have symptoms of abnormal bleeding such as easy bruising. When the Factor VIII level is less than 1% of normal then the condition is classified as severe.

The management of patients with haemophilia who are to undergo surgery relies on a threefold regimen. Therapy can:
• Increase Factor VIII production
• Replace missing Factor VIII
• Inhibit fibrinolysis.

Factor VIII levels can be increased by 1-desamino-8-D-arginine vasopressin (DDAVP). In patients with mild forms of the disease this therapy may be sufficient; it may be supplemented with an antifibrinolytic agent (see below) in others.

Replacement therapy is with cryoprecipitate, Factor VIII, fresh frozen plasma or purified forms of Factor VIII. Unfortunately some individuals

with haemophilia produce Factor VIII inhibitors. In some cases the level of inhibitors is low and can be combated with high doses of Factor VIII. However, in others the inhibitors are induced in response to Factor VIII and this represents a problem. Inhibitors may be overcome by administering activated Factor IX or prothrombin complex concentrates.

Antifibrinolytic therapy is useful in the post-surgical phase to protect the formed blood clot. Agents used in this way include tranexamic acid and epsilon-amino caproic acid (EACA).

Christmas disease is not as common as haemophilia but is similar to the latter condition with the exception that the problem is reduced Factor IX action. Management is the same as with Haemophilia A except that any replacement therapy is with Factor IX that is not present in cryoprecipitate.

As with haemophilia von Willebrand's disease has variable severity. This condition is not sex-linked and is more common than haemophilia. The disease presents with prolonged bleeding times and reduced factor VIII activity. In mild cases DDAVP and anti-fibrinolytic therapy are sufficient to cover surgical procedures. However, in severe cases Factor VIII replacement therapy is required.

As well as problems with bleeding these patients may be infected with HIV or hepatitis viruses because of the transfusion of infected blood or blood products.

In addition to congenital causes, problems with clotting may arise due to liver disease or because of drug therapy. An example is the patient who abuses alcohol. Before performing surgery on patients with potential liver problems it is essential to perform a clotting screen to determine if any corrective therapy must be provided to achieve good haemostasis.

Drugs that interfere with clotting include warfarin and heparin. The management of patients on these medications is discussed below.

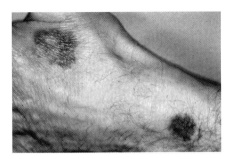

Fig. 4 Bruising on the hand should alert the dentist to a bleeding problem

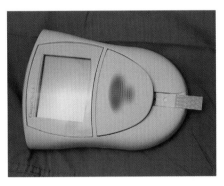

Fig. 5 The INR can be measured at the chair side by portable machines that require only a finger-prick blood sample

VASCULAR PROBLEMS

An example of a vascular disorder is hereditary haemorrhagic telangiectasia. Vascular defects due to deficiency states such as scurvy are rare nowadays, except in some members of immigrant communities. Vascular problems encountered are mainly the result of immunological or connective tissue disease (such as Ehler's- Danlos syndrome). Patients with vascular disorders have a prolonged bleeding time. Local haemostatic measures are all that are usually employed to arrest haemorrhage.

FIBRINOLYTIC PROBLEMS

Problems with fibrinolysis are not commonly encountered in dental practice. This effect can be produced by drugs (eg streptokinase used as a 'clot-buster' to treat thromboses or pulmonary embolism) or by disease. Plasmin levels may be increased in hepatic or malignant disease such as prostate carcinoma. The treatment is to use an antifibrinolytic agent such as tranexamic acid which is prescribed in hospital practice but is not available for use in the dental practice.

EXAMINATION

Anaemia may be obvious as pallor of the skin and mucosa but this can be rather subjective. A glossitis may be due to deficiency anaemia. Opportunistic infections or oral ulceration may indicate defects in red or white cells. Gingival enlargement or bleeding, oral paraesthesia or swellings of the parotid glands may be presenting signs of leukaemia. Signs of bleeding disorders may be apparent during the general assessment of the patient prior to intra-oral examination. Jaundice may be present indicating hepatic disease that can result in clotting problems. Bruising or petechiae on the arms and hands may be visible (*Fig. 4*). There may also be signs of bruising intra-orally, especially in areas subjected to trauma from the dentition or a denture. Bleeding gingiva in the absence of inflammatory periodontal disease should raise the level of suspicion.

INFLUENCE OF HAEMATOLOGICAL AND BLEEDING DISORDERS ON DENTAL MANAGEMENT

The management of patients with haematological and bleeding disorders in dentistry may be complex. The following aspects must be considered.
1. Surgical procedures
2. Choice of anaesthesia
3. Medication prescribed
4. Cross-infection control.

Surgical procedures

Healing after surgical procedures may be compromised in patients with anaemia or white cell disorders and antibiotics should be administered if this is a concern. The aim is to achieve optimum levels of antibiotic in the forming blood clot so they must be given prophylactically,[2] not after the procedure. Anaemia is not a contra-indication to the provision of minor surgical procedures in dental practice.

The timing of surgery in patients undergoing treatment for conditions such as leukaemia is important. Surgical treatments should be performed during stages of remission and between chemotherapeutic regimens when the cell count is optimal. Close liaison with the supervising haematologist is vital.

No surgical procedure, no matter how minor, should be performed on a patient with a bleeding disorder without prior consultation with the patient's haematologist or physician. Patients with congenital bleeding disorders should be treated in specialist centres where co-operation between surgeon and haematologist is established. Patients with haemophilia A, Christmas disease or von Willebrand's disease may require replacement therapy prior to surgery and an antifibrinolytic agent post-operatively. The use of local measures such as suturing and packing with a haemostatic agent should also be considered to prevent post-operative haemorrhage (*Figs 2 and 3*).

The management of patients taking drugs that interfere with bleeding is controversial. If aspirin needs to be withdrawn then therapy should cease 10 days before surgery as the effect of the drug on platelets is irreversible and replacement of the platelet population will take this length of time to occur. However, aspirin therapy does not normally need to be stopped and local haemostatic measures normally suffice. Similarly other antiplatelet drugs such as clopidogrel and dipyridamole do not need to be stopped prior to surgery and local measures control bleeding. These patients can receive minor surgical procedures in general practice.

Patients taking warfarin should have their INR (International Normalised Ratio – a measure of the prothrombin time) measured prior to any surgical procedure. This can now be performed at the chair-side with a finger-prick sample (*Fig. 5*). The normal therapeutic INR for patients on warfarin is 2.0 to 3.0 except for those with cardiac valve replacement where the range is 2.5-3.5. A level above 4.0 is non-therapeutic and requires adjustment of the warfarin dose. One question that has to be addressed is whether it is more dangerous to reduce the level of anticoagulation with the risk of a thrombo-embolic episode than to

perform surgery in the warfarinised patient. There is evidence that patients are more likely to die from a thrombo-embolic problem than they are to develop a bleed that does not settle with local haemostatic measures.[3]

Current opinion[4,5] is that most surgical operations that can be performed in dental practice such as extractions and simple minor oral surgical procedures may be carried out if the INR is less than 4.0 without alteration of the warfarin dosage. If the INR is greater than 4.0 referral to the supervising physician is needed. If possible deep regional block anaesthesia should be avoided, for example by the use of intraligamentary injections in the mandible. Post-operative bleeding should be controlled by local measures such as suturing haemostatic packs.

Patients receiving heparin will not be encountered regularly in dental practice. Those who may seek treatment are patients on haemodialysis due to renal failure. These patients are heparinised on the days they are dialysed (normally 3 alternate days a week). However, due to the short half-life of heparin (around 5 hours) the effect is short-lived and treatment can be performed safely on the days between dialysis.

Choice of anaesthesia

Anaemia should be corrected before intravenous sedation or general anaesthesia as the reduction in oxygen carrying capacity could be dangerous. The use of nitrous oxide sedation is probably best avoided in patients with pernicious anaemia, as one of the side effects of this gas is the production of vitamin B_{12} deficiency.[6]

The concern for patients with bleeding disorders is local anaesthesia. The use of deep injections such as inferior alveolar nerve blocks is contra-indicated in patients with bleeding problems unless some form of prophylaxis has been provided. This is for fear of producing a bleed that may track around the pharynx leading to airway obstruction. Fortunately there are alternative methods of anaesthetising mandibular teeth, which allow this problem to be circumvented. Haemophiliac patients who had received intraligamentary anaesthesia for restorative dentistry without administration of Factor VIII recorded no complications related to haemorrhage or haematoma formation.[7,8] Infiltration injections should not produce significant problems.

Medication prescribed

A number of drugs that dentists may prescribe can interfere with haemorrhage control and cause bleeding; the classic example is aspirin, which interferes with platelet function as described above. In addition, some drugs commonly used in dentistry including analgesics and antimicrobials interact with anticoagulants. Aspirin, diclofenac, diflunisal, ibuprofen and prolonged use of paracetamol all increase the effect of warfarin. Penicillins can increase the prothrombin time when given to patients receiving warfarin. However this effect is uncommon. Erythromycin enhances the anti-coagulant effects of both warfarin and nicoumalone by reducing the metabolism of the latter drugs. Combined use is not absolutely contra-indicated but monitoring of the patient is required. The effect of warfarin is significantly increased by metronidazole due to the antibiotic inhibiting the metabolism of the anticoagulant. This interaction is clinically important.[9] If metronidazole is essential then the dose of warfarin may have to be reduced. Tetracycline may enhance the anticoagulant effect of warfarin and the other coumarin anticoagulants. Miconazole enhances the anti-coagulant effect of warfarin even after topical use. Dentists should know about this important interaction as it may lead to catastrophic bleeding. A case has been reported of a warfarinised patient's INR increasing from 2.5 to 17.9 following the use of miconazole oral gel.[10] One other drug worth mentioning is carbamazepine. This may reduce the effect of warfarin due to increased metabolism of the anti-coagulant.

Cross-infection control

The chances of transmitting infected material between patients or from patient to operator should be minimised for all dental treatments. However, this is especially so when treating patients who are at high risk of carrying viral diseases such as HIV and hepatitis. Sadly some patients who have received treatments for bleeding disorders, principally multiple transfusions of blood products, fall into this category. Rigorous cross-infection control measures must be adopted when dealing with these patients.

CONCLUSIONS

Haematological problems impact on all aspects of dentistry. The taking of a thorough history and close liaison with medical colleagues will help reduce the problems that may occur in the patient with disorders of the blood. Patients with clotting defects represent a challenge to both surgical and restorative dentistry. Although all patients should have their management discussed with their supervising haematologist or physician when surgical procedures are to be performed, many cases can be adequately treated using local measures and skills commonly employed by dentists.

1. Seymour R A, Meechan J G, Walton J G. *Adverse Drug Reactions in Dentistry 2nd ed.* pp 140 – 142. Oxford: Oxford University Press, 1996.
2. Peterson L J. Antibiotic prophylaxis against wound infections in oral and maxillofacial surgery. *J Oral Maxillofac Surg* 1990; **48:** 617-620.
3. Wahl M J. Myths of dental surgery in patients receiving anticoagulant therapy. *J Am Dent Assoc* 2000; **131:** 77-81.
4. Surgical management of the primary care dental patient on warfarin. North West Medicines Information Centre, 70 Pembroke Place, Liverpool, 2001.
5. British Committee for Standards in Haematology. Guidelines for the management of patients on oral anticoagulants requiring dental surgery. Online at http://www.bcshguidelines.com/pdf/warfarinandoralsurgery26407.pdf.
6. Donaldson D, Meechan J G. The hazards of chronic exposure to nitrous oxide. An update. *Br Dent J* 1995; **178:** 95-100.
7. Ah Pin P J. The use of intraligamental injections in haemophiliacs. *Br. Dent. J.* 1987;**162:** 151-152.
8. Spuller R L. Use of the periodontal ligamentary injection in dental care of the patient with haemophilia - a clinical evaluation. *Spec Care Dent* 1988; **8:** 28-29.
9. Kazmier F J. A significant interaction between metronidazole and warfarin. *Mayo Clin Proc* 1987; **51:** 782-784.
10. Colquhoun M C, Daly M, Stewart P, Beeley L. Interaction between warfarin and miconazole oral gel. *Lancet* 1987; **i:** 695-696.

Chapter 10
The paediatric patient

M. Greenwood, J. G. Meechan and R. R. Welbury*

*Professor of Paediatric Dentistry, University of Glasgow

IN BRIEF

- Disease can affect dental development in children
- Congenital conditions can interfere with provision of dental treatment
- Underlying disease and its treatment can affect the timing of dental treatment in children
- Diseases of childhood influence the choice of anaesthesia
- Close co-operation with paediatricians is important in managing children with serious conditions
- Liaison is needed not neglect

Medical problems in children can cause unique difficulties for the safe provision of dental treatment.[1] Such problems can affect the type and timing of dental treatment as well as methods of control of pain and anxiety. In this chapter conditions which influence the choice of anaesthesia as well as those which affect dental development are discussed.

POINTS IN THE HISTORY

Background information

Some conditions are relevant since they affect oral and dental development and will often be discovered in a thorough history. These include disorders of bone such as cleidocranial dysplasia where delayed eruption and multiple supernumerary teeth occur and fibrous dysplasia which can produce malocclusions (see Chapter 8). Disorders localised to the teeth such as amelogenesis imperfecta provide a challenge to preventive and restorative dentistry. Other disorders such as dentinogenesis imperfecta may be associated with osteogenesis imperfecta and

surgery may be hazardous. Referral to an oral surgeon is sensible in such cases. Hypodontia[2] occurs in ectodermal dysplasia and successful management of this condition often requires co-ordinated specialist treatment. The general dental practitioner, however, has an important role in the management of these patients.

The medical history in a child patient should follow a similar theme to that of an adult but there are differences in emphasis in certain areas. It is useful to obtain information regarding previous levels of compliance with treatment since disorders that interfere with patient co-operation can make routine dental treatment difficult. Conditions such as severe physical and mental disability, severe convulsive disorders and extensive behavioural problems can create problems. Techniques such as relative analgesia (RA) can be used with success in some of these patients but there are limits to what can be achieved since a level of co-operation and understanding is required.

Organ transplantation is a procedure which is relatively commonplace today and the number of children with renal, heart, heart/lung, liver and bone transplants will increase. The dental team can play an important role in pre-transplant assessment as it is vital that any focus of infection is eliminated prior to transplantation.

Disorders of different organ systems have been described in the earlier chapters in this book. Problems that impact on the younger patient are discussed more fully here.

Cardiovascular conditions

Close consultation with the cardiologist is required if a cardiac condition is encountered, particularly if there is functional limitation.

The patient may have Down Syndrome (trisomy 21). This occurs in 1 in 700 live births. In nearly half of Down's patients, congenital cardiac anomalies are found. There is some degree of learning disability in all these patients and immunological defects predispose them to infection. Down's patients have a higher risk of developing acute leukaemia than the general population.

Respiratory conditions

Asthma affects about 12% of all children. The severity varies from mild to moderate to severe. In mild cases attacks are only occasional and can be precipitated by infection. Between attacks patients are asymptomatic. In moderate cases episodes are severe and recurrent but patients are symptom-free between attacks. Exercise induces bronchoconstriction. When a child suffers from severe asthma, attacks vary in severity but the child is never asymptomatic and the illness affects growth and lung function. A history should always ascertain the degree of severity of the asthma and the efficacy of prescribed treatment.

Cystic fibrosis is an inherited disorder of exocrine glands. It occurs in 1 in 2000 births and is inherited as autosomal recessive. Mucus has an increased viscosity and pancreatic insufficiency in childhood occurs. Diabetes mellitus may be a complication and some patients have cirrhosis of the liver. Recurrent respiratory infections may occur resulting in bronchiectasis.

Haematological conditions

Disorders such as anaemia and leukaemia, in addition to interfering with wound healing may also lead to a bleeding tendency and consultation with the haematologist or oncologist is essential before considering surgery on such children.

It is important to enquire about Sickle-cell disease in patients of African, Asian and West Indian descent since the administration of a general anaesthetic to an undiagnosed sufferer can cause severe complications. Deoxygenation during anaesthesia causes the erythrocyte to deform into a sickle shape which causes the cells to aggregate and inhibits blood flow in small diameter vessels. A finger prick Sickledex test, if positive should be followed by haemoglobin electrophoresis. In patients of Mediterranean descent, the possibility of thalassaemia should be borne in mind.

It is important to enquire about possible bleeding disorders. Congenital disorders such as haemophilia and acquired clotting disorders preclude surgical dental treatment outside the hospital environment. The most common hereditary haemophilias (sex-linked recessive) are Haemophilia A (Factor VIII deficiency) and Haemophilia B (Factor IX deficiency). These patients require replacement of the appropriate clotting factor(s) prior to surgery and usually the provision of anti-fibrinolytic therapy following treatment. Treatment planning and timing of intervention must be co-ordinated with the haematologist. Children with platelet deficiencies (*Fig. 1*) may require a platelet transfusion or if the problem is one of idiopathic thrombocytopaenic purpura then a pre-operative course of steroids can increase platelet numbers to an acceptable level for surgery (greater than 50×10^9 per litre).

Neurological conditions

Enquiry should be made about any history of convulsions since the stress of dentistry may induce fits in epileptic patients. Epilepsy affects 3-5% of the paediatric population and most cases are idiopathic. Attacks may be stimulated by hyperventilation, fever, photic stimulation, withdrawal of anticonvulsants (or poor compliance), lack of sleep, over sedation, over hydration, emotional upset and some medications eg antihistamines. The use of relative analgesia can be of great benefit for children with a history of convulsions in the dental chair.

Cerebral palsy is the leading cause of significant disability in children. Uncontrolled movement and abnormal posture are the main handicaps but other neurological and mental problems can also occur. Epilepsy, visual and hearing impairment are features which may cause difficulties with dental treatment.

A number of children with hydrocephalus have shunts which drain cerebrospinal fluid (CSF) from the brain to other areas of the body thereby reducing intracranial pressure and preventing brain damage. An older form of shunt drained fluid from the brain to the ventricles of the heart (atrio-ventricular). A newer shunt drains fluid to the peritoneum (atrio-peritoneal).

Renal conditions

Renal disease in children mainly comprises the so-called nephritic syndromes which may progress to chronic kidney disease (CKD). Progression to CKD leads to the need for dialysis and possibly transplantation. CKD patients may cause difficulties with management due to corticosteroid and other immunosuppression therapy. Potential problems include:

- Impaired drug excretion
- Anaemia
- Bleeding tendencies
- Associated anticoagulant therapy
- Hypertension
- Infections e.g. hepatitis B
- Renal osteodystrophy.

Hepatic conditions

Chronic liver disease with impaired hepatic function is uncommon in childhood (*Fig. 2*). Problems can be categorised into:
- Coagulation disorders
- Drug toxicity
- Disorders of fluid and electrolyte balance
- Problems with drug therapy
- Infections.

Endocrine conditions

Insulin-controlled diabetic children who require a general anaesthetic should be treated as in-patients because the starvation required before the procedure would render them hypoglycaemic. Hospitalisation will enable them to be stabilised pre- and post-operatively on an intravenous drip that will control both sugar and insulin. There is no contraindication to treatment in general dental practice under local anaesthetic or local anaesthetic with IS as long as the treatment time does not interfere with a normal snack intake. Extra carbohydrate can always be taken in liquid form prior to a procedure.

Drug therapy

Although there have been positive moves towards the provision of sugar-free medication[3,4] there are still cases of dental caries exacerbated by drug therapy (*Fig. 3*). This can be due either to the direct effect of sugar-based medicines or by an indirect action such as xerostomia. Medications which can produce xerostomia in children include antihistamines and major tranquillisers.

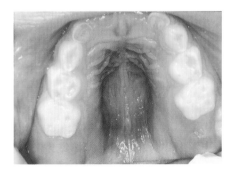

Fig. 1 A palatal bruise in a child taking immunosuppressants. This has lead to a low platelet count

Table 1 Points in the history in a paediatric patient
• Previous levels of compliance with treatment • Asthma • Diabetes • Cystic Fibrosis • Sickle Cell Disease • Thalassaemia • Bleeding disorders • Epilepsy • Shunt in hydrocephalus • Cranio-facial disorders • Renal disorders • Hepatic conditions • Drug therapy

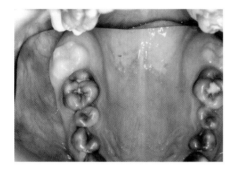

Fig. 2 Severely bilirubin stained teeth that started mineralising pre-liver transplant at age 2.5 years. The second permanent molars are normal

A summary of salient points in the history of a child dental patient are shown in *Table 1*. It should not be forgotten that abuse of drugs during pregnancy can produce oro-facial defects in children. For example, cleft lip and palate are seen in the foetal alcohol syndrome and cigarette smoking can cause reduction in crown size of primary teeth. Cocaine misuse by mothers has been associated with tongue-tie in their offspring.[5]

Craniofacial disorders

Certain inherited or acquired craniofacial disorders eg temporomandibular joint ankylosis, should be enquired about since access to the mouth may be limited causing difficulties with treatment. In some cases surgical correction of the deformity is necessary before intra-oral procedures can be performed.

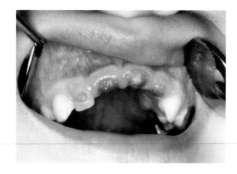

Fig. 3 Caries due to prolonged use of sweetened liquid oral medicines

EXAMINATION

The degree to which it will be possible to achieve compliance with dental treatment can be obvious very quickly in a consultation. The child may have a condition that interferes with their ability to co-operate.

In cleidocranial dysplasia there may be delayed eruption and multiple supernumerary teeth whilst in fibrous dysplasia and cerebral palsy a malocclusion may be present as mentioned earlier. The disorder may specifically affect the teeth eg amelogenesis imperfecta or a systemic condition may be associated with an abnormal dentition. Dentinogenesis imperfecta may be associated with osteogenesis imperfecta or hypodontia with ectodermal dysplasia. There may in addition be extensive caries that has been exacerbated by drug therapy.

Patients with Down syndrome tend to have an open mouthed posture with a protruding tongue which can cause difficulties with dental treatment. Tooth development and eruption is retarded. An anterior open bite is common, as is a class III malocclusion. The incidence of cleft lip and palate is increased in these patients. Periodontal disease is severe and has an early onset but caries incidence, by comparison, is surprisingly low.

In cystic fibrosis there are recurrent chest infections and often a productive cough. Many patients also have nasal polyps and recurrent sinusitis which may preclude the use of RA due to the poor nasal airway. The salivary glands may be enlarged. The enamel may be hypoplastic and eruption dates may be delayed. Medication may produce

oral signs, for example the pancreatic replacement drug pancreatin may produce oral ulceration.

The possibility of child abuse is an important phenomenon which should always be borne in mind if findings on examination appear to be inconsistent with the history. An injury where there has been a long delay between the incident and attendance for treatment is a cause for suspicion. Injuries which do not 'fit' with the history and multiple injuries, particularly those which appear to be of different ages are also cause for concern. Child abuse, whilst more common in the lower social classes, is by no means confined to these groups. Local area Child Protection Committee Guidelines will be available to guide the dental practitioner in their referral.

GENERAL AND LOCAL ANAESTHESIA, SEDATION AND MANAGEMENT CONSIDERATIONS IN THE PAEDIATRIC DENTAL PATIENT

The possibility of local anaesthetic toxicity is more likely in children than adults due to their smaller size. A dose of 1/10th of a cartridge per kilogram as a maximum is recommended,[6] this means that two cartridges is the maximum in a healthy 20kg 5-year-old. The use of local anaesthetics should be reduced in children with liver disorders. The use of any drug, including local anaesthetics in children with severe hepatic dysfunction should be discussed with the supervising physician. The use of local anaesthetics containing vasoconstrictors eg adrenaline should be avoided when injecting into an area with a compromised blood supply such as a mandible which has been irradiated for the treatment of childhood malignancy. Intraligamentary and infiltraton anaesthesia are the techniques of choicein the mandible for children with bleeding disorders such as haemophilia when restorative dental treatment is required.

In patients with sickle cell disease, if practicable, LA with or without RA is preferable to GA. If a GA is required in a patient with the sickle trait, careful oxygenation must be ensured. Patients with the disease itself may need a pre-anaesthetic transfusion so that the level of haemoglobin A is at least 50%.

The use of transcutaneous electronic nerve stimulation has been shown to be effective in reducing injection discomfort in children,[7] however this should be avoided in epileptic children and those with cardiac pacemakers.

Children with mild or moderate asthma, if asymptomatic at the time of treatment, do not need prophylaxis pre-treatment. If oral medication is being taken, this should be continued to prevent rebound bronchospasm. If the asthma is severe there is greater risk of bronchospasm being induced by GA or the stress of surgery. If GA is required the child must be in optimal condition ie no evidence of respiratory infection and an in-patient facility should be available.

In children with cystic fibrosis, sputum clearance is assisted by regular physiotherapy. Amoxycillin or flucloxacillin are used (often long-term) as prophylaxis against chest infection. If respiratory function is poor, GA is contra-indicated. Tetracycline, which is a very effective broad spectrum antibiotic may need to be given when children develop multiple drug sensitivity.

Diabetes and cirrhosis can also cause difficulties with dental treatment provision. In children with diabetes, infections and surgical procedures which create stress or alter food intake may disturb diabetic control. Diabetic children are best managed under LA if possible. Any infection should be treated vigorously. In children with cirrhosis, routine dental treatment is not usually a problem. A physician should be consulted if GA or surgery is needed due to the possibility of bleeding tendency, anaemia and the possibility of drug toxicity.

Intravenous sedation is considered unsuitable for children as it is unpredictable. Inhalation sedation (IS) is the technique of choice. IS has been shown to be an acceptable and cost-effective alternative to general anaesthesia in children having minor oral surgery.[8] The contra-indications to the use of IS include respiratory disorders. Acute upper respiratory tract infections necessitate postponement of treatment whereas chronic obstructive pulmonary disease is an absolute contra-indication. Children who suffer from myasthenia gravis should not be treated with IS outside a hospital environment since they are at risk of respiratory arrest and even in the hospital setting consultation with the physician is essential before considering anything other than local anaesthesia. Children with severe behavioural problems and those who suffer from claustrophobia are not suited to IS as they may not be able to tolerate the nasal mask. Certain surgical procedures in children, such as labial fraenectomy, are not possible under IS as the mask denies access to the surgical site.

Oral sedation is not in widespread use for children in the UK to facilitate dental treatment. As with any other drug, allergy to an oral sedative obviously precludes its use. Drugs which are used in the U.K. include benzodiazepines, chloral hydrate derivatives and promethazine. Hepatic or renal impairment is a contra-indication to use of outpatient oral sedation. Similarly the concurrent administration of any central nervous system depressant prevents the use of oral sedation. In addition, chloral hydrate derivatives and promethazine should be avoided in the presence of cardiovascular disease.

In patients with Down syndrome the possibility of cardiac anomalies should be borne in mind. Immunological impairment means that respiratory infections are more likely and there may additional congenital abnormalities of the respiratory tract. The hypoplastic mid-face may cause difficulties with endotracheal intubation. General anaesthesia may also be complicated by the possibility of atlanto-axial subluxation when extending the neck if care is not taken. These patients, when institutionalised, have increased likelihood of hepatitis B carriage.

Children who have disorders likely to adversely affect wound healing should be treated with prophylactic antibiotics. These include children with decreased resistance to infection. Metabolic disturbances such as uncontrolled diabetes and long-term use of corticosteroids also affect wound healing. Well controlled diabetic patients should be considered 'normal' in relation to healing. Haematological problems such as anaemia, leukaemia and cyclic neutropaenia also affect healing ability. Children on immunosuppressant therapy and those being treated with anti-metabolites or local irradiation are also at risk of post-surgical infection. The objective of prophylactic use of antibiotics is to achieve optimal drug concentration in the initial blood clot. Timing of antibiotic administration is aimed at having optimal blood levels of the antimicrobial at the end of the surgical procedure (ie when the clot forms). Consultation with the supervising paediatrician is essential prior to the use of antibiotics in children with significant renal or hepatic impairment.

The use of anti-metabolites to treat childhood malignancies such as leukaemia is not a contra-indication to dental treatment but it does affect its timing. Consultation with the appropriate paediatrician is again important here in order that essential treatment can be performed at the optimal time during cyclical anti-cancer therapy when platelet and white cell counts are acceptable. This treatment is best completed in a hospital setting whilst the patient is undergoing chemotherapy.[9]

The production of a healthy mouth should be the 'accepted norm' before transplant surgery and consultation with the transplant team and physicians is essential to determine the influence of the organ deficit on dental treatment. The transplanted heart reacts differently to the normal heart to epinephrine.[10] This is apparent after the use of epinephrine-containing dental local anaesthetics.[11] It is sensible to use dose reductions or even avoid use of this vasoconstrictor in the child who has had a cardiac transplant. The management of all transplant patients is complicated by maintenance drug therapy. Steroid therapy may necessitate the administration of a steroid boost prior to stressful procedures and the possibility of adrenal crisis must be borne in mind. The use of post-transplant immunosuppressant therapy can increase the risk of haemorrhage and post-surgical infection. Post-transplantation therapy with drugs such as ciclosporin and nifedipine leads to gingival overgrowth similar to that seen with epanutin. Regular oral hygiene review is essential and repeated surgical visits for gingival recontouring may well be required.

CONCLUSIONS

Advances in medical care (especially in the treatment of childhood malignancy and organ transplantation) mean that dentists are increasingly likely to encounter medically compromised children. The keys to successful treatment are:

- Accurate medical history
- Close liaison with medical colleagues and not neglect
- Rigorous preventative programmes
- Dental intervention at times appropriate to medical care
- Regular follow-up.

1. Shaw L S. Medically compromised children. In: Paediatric Dentistry. (3rd ed) Ed R.R. Welbury, M. S. Duggal and M-T Hosie. Oxford: Oxford University Press, 2005.
2. Hobkirk J A, Goodman J R, Jones S P. Presenting complaints and findings in a group of patients attending a hypodontia clinic. *Br Dent J* 1994; **177:** 337- 339
3. British National Formulary available online at http://bnf.org.
4. Maguire A, Evans D J, Rugg-Gunn A J, Butler T J. Evaluation of sugar-free medicines campaign in north-east England: quantitative analysis of medicines use. *Comm Dent Health* 1999; **16:** 138-144.
5. Harris E F, Friend G W, Toley E A. Enhanced prevalence of ankyloglossia with maternal cocaine use. *Cleft Pal Craniofac J* 1992; **29:** 72-76.
6. Meechan J G. How to avoid local anaesthetic toxicity. *Br Dent J* 1998; **184:** 334- 335.
7. Wilson S, Molina L de L, Preisch J, Weaver J. The effect of electronic dental anesthesia on behaviour during local anesthetic injection in the young, sedated dental patient. *Paediatic Dent* 1999; **21:** 12-7.
8. Shaw A, Meechan J G, Kilpatrick N, Welbury R R. The use of inhalation sedation and local anaesthesia instead of general anaesthesia for extractions and minor oral surgery in children: a prospective study. *Int J Paed Dent* 1996; **6:** 7- 11.
9. Fayle S A, Duggal M S, Williams S A. Oral problems and the dentist's role in the management of paediatric oncology patients. *Dent Update* 1992;May 152-159.
10. Gilbert E M, Eiswirht C C, Mealey P C, Larrabee B S, Herrick C M, Bristow MR. β -adrenergic supersensitivity of the transplanted human heart is presynaptic in origin. *Circulation* 1989; **79:** 344-349.
11. Meechan J G, Parry G, Rattray D T, Thomason J M. Effects of Dental Local Anaesthetics in Cardiac Transplant Recipients. *Br Dent J* 2002; **192** 161-163.

Chapter 11
The older patient

M. Greenwood, R. H. Jay and J. G. Meechan

IN BRIEF

- Frail older people require special consideration in order to successfully receive the healthcare they require.
- Older people often suffer with multiple medical problems and are taking multiple medications.
- Physical disability, impaired vision and hearing and reduced mental function cause practical difficulties.
- Liaison with the patient's carers and general medical practitioner is vital.

The proportion of older people in the UK population has been on the increase for several years. Dental practitioners who treat the general public often see older patients on a regular basis. This chapter considers aspects of clinical management in the older patient with particular reference to the presentation of disease and factors to be considered in prescribing medication.

INTRODUCTION

A significant proportion of any general dentist's work will be with those over retiring age, but it is the over 80 age group that has the largest population growth rate, and which often presents with multiple ongoing medical problems requiring multiple medications, and with disabilities requiring special consideration.

POINTS IN THE HISTORY

One definition of ageing is 'the gradual development of changes in structure and function that are not due to preventable disease or trauma, and that are associated with decreased functional capacity and an increased probability of death'. Although this definition of the pure ageing process excludes age-related disease, older people suffer from a wide range of medical conditions and accumulate long term consequences of past illnesses. Some common medical problems of old age are listed in *Table 1*.

It is essential to know an older person's medical background when assessing or treating any new health problem. Many of the conditions listed in *Table 1* have a direct effect on the delivery of dental treatment. To take the example of common cardiovascular disorders, in patients with ischaemic heart disease, angina may be brought on by the stress of dental treatment, and may need to be treated in the surgery with sublingual nitrates. Lying flat may aggravate breathlessness in heart failure patients. Those with atrial fibrillation are likely to be on anticoagulants, and may have ischaemic heart disease, heart failure or underlying valvular conditions.

Table 2 lists certain features which distinguish illness in older people from that in the younger population. Older people often present with atypical symptoms, or nonspecific presentations of disease. For example, loss

Table 1 Common medical conditions of old age
Cardiovascular
- Ischaemic heart disease – angina/myocardial infarction - Heart failure - Atrial fibrillation
Respiratory
- Chronic obstructive pulmonary disease (COPD) - Respiratory infections
Gastrointestinal
- Gastro-oesophageal reflux - Peptic ulceration - Constipation
Genitourinary
- Incontinence - Urine frequency - Obstructive uropathy due to prostate disease
Musculoskeletal
- Arthritis - Osteoporosis and fractures - Muscle weakness
Neurological/Psychiatric
- Poor vision - Deafness - Poor memory/confusion/dementia - Depression/agitation/anxiety - Parkinson's disease - Strokes
Metabolic/Endocrine
- Diabetes mellitus (type 2, non-insulin-dependent) - Hypothyroidism
Neoplastic
- Common cancers in old age include breast, lung, gastrointestinal tract and prostate.

of appetite and weight may have many potential causes including physical illness such as cancer, mental illnesses including depression, and oral conditions. It is therefore important to obtain as clear a picture as possible of the presenting complaint.

The adverse effects of ageing and illness on functional ability result in the so-called 'giants of geriatric medicine', listed in *Table 3*. They all have obvious practical consequences for the delivery of dental care, and the practitioner should enquire whether any special consideration needs to be given, for example assistance with mobility or toilet use.

A commonly-used framework of headings for taking a medical history is given in *Table 4*. Obtaining a clear and full history from an older person can be difficult. The complexity of their medical history itself may result in omission or misunderstanding on the patient's part. Communication may be impeded by visual impairment or deafness. The patient may suffer from impaired memory, poor concentration or frank dementia. Therefore, it is important to recognise these problems, seek a corroborative history from a relative or carer, and to confirm medical details with the patient's general medical practitioner.

Since illness is often associated with loss of function or independence, it is important to enquire about the impact of the condition on the patient's life. This may often be quite disproportionate to the apparent seriousness of the underlying condition. For example, a relatively minor oral infection in a frail older person may result in the person stopping eating and drinking, becoming dehydrated and consequently requiring emergency hospital admission. Conversely, the older person's stoicism and expectations of ill health can sometimes result in late presentation of advanced disease, the symptoms of which had wrongly been accepted as a natural consequence of old age.

Social circumstances and support are important considerations for older people with reduced physical or mental function. The ability to co-operate

with aspects of dental treatment such as maintaining oral hygiene or taking prescribed medication may be impaired. Aids and appliances can significantly enhance an older person's independence with activities of daily living. Written instructions and reminders may be helpful in those with impaired memory. Actual physical help or supervision from a carer is needed when other measures fail. It is therefore essential to ascertain details of the support that is available to the patient, for example whether they live with an able relative, have carers visiting them in their home, or live in a protected institution with 24 hour care. Over 20% of those over 85 years of age will live in a residential or nursing home or sheltered housing.

Drug-related problems are common in older people. Compliance is often poor, and the list of medications provided by the general medical practitioner may differ significantly from what the patient is actually taking. Therefore, obtaining a correct drug history often requires effort beyond simply transcribing a list from the GMP, or asking the patient what they take. Checking through a prescription list with the patient and their carer and reading the labels of medications or dosing boxes brought by the patient are valuable ways of obtaining correct information.

EXAMINATION OF THE OLDER DENTAL PATIENT

Specific points in the examination of patients with the medical conditions listed in *Table 1* have been covered in chapters 1-9. This chapter will therefore concentrate on the more general features in older people, and assessment of their function and ability.

An idea of an older person's physical function can be obtained by general observation. Do they appear well-nourished? Is their gait strong and steady, or do they use walking aids? Do they appear breathless on walking? Are there obvious bone or joint deformities from arthritis or osteoporotic fracture? How good is their manual dexterity when removing

Table 2 Features of illness in older people

- Nonspecific presentation
- Multiple pathology and consequent polypharmacy
- Interaction between conditions and between medications
- Loss of functional independence
- Impaired homeostasis, resistance to disease and recovery.

Table 3 Giants of geriatric medicine

- Incontinence
- Instability (falls)
- Immobility
- Intellectual impairment (dementia and delirium).

Table 4 Elements of a medical history

- Presenting complaint
- History of presenting complaint
- Past history (including ongoing chronic problems)
- Review of other systems
- Family history
- Social history
- Treatment history – drugs and allergies.

their coat or signing forms? Can they see and hear adequately?

Observation may be used to deduce the mental function of elderly patients informally. Do they appear orientated to their surroundings, able to concentrate and converse appropriately? Are they clean and appropriately dressed? Are their answers to questions clear and plausible?

There are pitfalls in the use of general observation, however. Apparent mental impairment in conversation may actually be due to deafness or a speech disorder such as dysphasia following a stroke. Conversely, a patient may be able to conceal significant dementia by maintaining social graces and giving plausible answers to questions.

Manual dexterity may be significantly impaired due to muscle weakness without obvious clues such as deforming arthritis or the tremor of Parkinson's disease. Patients with macular degeneration of the retina may have severely impaired central vision, to the level of being registered blind, while retaining sufficient peripheral vision for safe navigation while walking into the surgery. All of these can have practical consequences

Table 5 National Service Framework for older people[9]
Standard 1: rooting out age discrimination
'NHS services will be provided, regardless of age, on the basis of clinical need alone…'
Standard 2: person-centred care
'NHS and social care services treat older people as individuals and enable them to make choices about their own care'
Standard 8: the promotion of health and active life in older age
'The health and well-being of older people is promoted through a coordinated programme of action…'

for the ability to co-operate with dental treatment and oral hygiene instructions or comply with the taking of medication.

DENTAL MANAGEMENT OF THE OLDER PATIENT

Some important principles of management of both health and social care were set out in the National Service Framework for older people, a government document which sets standards of care in England and Wales.[1] Three standards relevant to dental care are given in *Table 5*.

An example of overt age discrimination found during work for standard 1 was a national guideline restricting conscious sedation for outpatient dental procedures to those less than 70 years of age. It is perfectly true that certain co-morbidities in older patients put them at increased risk of harm from sedation. It may cause respiratory suppression in patients with chronic lung disease, confusion in those with underlying chronic brain conditions or falls in those with postural instability. However, it is not appropriate to introduce such a generalisation for all patients over 70 receiving sedation. Certainly some elderly patients have the ability to appropriately cope with patient-controlled sedation.[2] Each case should be considered on its own merits, and provision made for inpatient treatment where sedation is warranted but increased risk is anticipated.

Covert age discrimination is also common, and can take three main forms.
- Health professionals may wrongly assume that an older person has a short life expectancy and therefore has limited capacity to benefit from certain interventions. The average life expectancy of an 80-year-old is 8 to 9 years[3]
- Services required by older people may be under-provided and have long waiting lists. The problem may be compounded if younger patients are given priority
- Services may be inconvenient or inaccessible to frail or disabled people who require assistance and transport. They may not know who to ask or how to seek the help required.

A key requirement for standard 2, relevant to dental healthcare, is the need to provide information available to older people in a way that they can understand. For the cognitively impaired, this may involve tolerant and careful explanation in simple language. For the visually impaired, information leaflets should be available in large print. Special effort is also needed to communicate effectively with hearing-impaired older people. When care is taken, the majority of older people can make appropriate choices and give valid consent. Where this is not possible, there is a duty to act in the patient's best interests and involve relatives and carers in decision making.

Standard 8 should contain dental health promotion, including screening programmes, routine checks and preventive treatment.

Dental problems commonly seen in the older patient are covered in other texts and will not be discussed here.

ADMINISTRATION OF MEDICINES AND PRESCRIBING FOR OLDER DENTAL PATIENTS

As older people are already taking multiple medications, there is increased likelihood of drug interactions. Their impaired homeostasis and multiple co-morbidities put them at increased risk of unwanted effects. It is therefore essential to take a full treatment history and document a patient's known medical conditions before prescribing.

Altered pharmacodynamics often increases the sensitivity of older people to drug actions. Renal function deteriorates with age, even in the absence of known renal disease, resulting in reduced drug excretion. Liver function also deteriorates, slowing elimination of drugs metabolised there. Low serum albumin in chronic ill health may increase free concentrations of protein-bound drugs. Absorption of drugs is often relatively normal, so the result of these changes is that older people often need lower doses, particularly of drugs with a narrow therapeutic window.

The most common drug that a dentist will prescribe to an elderly patient is a local anaesthetic. It is important not to overdose the elderly patient and this may happen more readily in this population compared to younger adults. This is the result of lower body weight (the maximum dose is determined by body weight) and also due to decreased ability to metabolise the drug. Most local anaesthetics are primarily metabolised in the liver and as hepatic function is decreased the chances of overdose increase. As a working rule it is sensible to halve the normal maximum dose in patients over 65 years of age.

As mentioned above, elderly patients may be taking a number of medications. The chance of an adverse reaction to local anaesthetics increases with medical risk factors.[4] A survey of local anaesthetic complications in Germany showed that the incidence of complications attributable to local anaesthesia in dentistry was 3.3% in patients with no risk factors compared to 6.9% in patients taking more than two medications daily.[4]

The anti-Parkinsonism drug entacapone is an inhibitor of the enzyme catechol-O-methyltransferase, which is the enzyme that initiates metabolism of exogenously administered adrenaline (such as during dental local anaesthesia). Thus, in patients taking this drug, dose-reduction or avoidance of adrenaline-containing local anaesthetics is advised.

It is not all bad news, however, in relation to local anaesthesia. There is evidence that the onset of local anaesthesia after intra-oral infiltration is more rapid in elderly patients compared to their younger counterparts.[5] In addition, the duration of pulpal anaesthesia may be longer in the older patient.[5] These effects on local anaesthesia may be the result of poorer vascularity and fatty degeneration of bone in the older patient.[5]

Of the medications listed in the Dental Practitioners' Formulary section of the British National Formulary,[6] most antibiotics can be prescribed at the standard doses. Some antibiotics and antifungals interact with warfarin, which older patients may be taking following cardiovascular disease or stroke and can be problematic. Single doses of drugs such as amoxicillin should not be troublesome but long term treatment with this antibiotic and metronidazole can alter clotting status, which is measured by the International Normalised Ratio (INR). Thus if these antibiotics are used, monitoring of the INR is required. The azole antifungal agents can cause dramatic increases in the INR, even topical use of miconazole can create this problem[7] and combined use is contraindicated. Many older patients take iron or calcium preparations, which can impair absorption of tetracyclines.

Non-steroidal anti-inflammatory drugs (NSAIDs) should be used with caution, particularly in patients with dyspepsia and those with renal disease or heart conditions requiring treatment with angiotensin converting enzyme (ACE) inhibitors and those taking anticoagulants. NSAIDs such as ibuprofen decrease the hypotensive effect of beta-blockers.

Older patients are particularly prone to side effects from drugs acting on the central nervous system, which can cause confusion, drowsiness and falls. This is especially true of benzodiazepines and other sedatives such as promethazine, but can also be a problem with opioid analgesics including pethidine.

Difficulty in dealing with multiple medications in the context of impaired vision, mental function or dexterity results in poor compliance. It is therefore important to consider means of enabling the patient to take their medication correctly. Careful explanation of the reason for the drug should be given, including whether it is 'as required' or to be taken as prescribed. It is useful to write down the main points and to explain them to a relative or carer. Small print on bottle labels may be difficult to read for the visually impaired patient, and childproof containers should be avoided unless the patient indicates that they are confident in their use. It may be difficult for the older patient with impaired manual dexterity to correctly dose liquid medicines if these have to be measured out using a spoon. One way round this problem is to provide a plastic syringe for drug dosing and dispensation.

Other means of enhancing compliance include supervision by a carer and the use of dosing boxes. These contain the medications set out in compartments labelled with the time and day of the week. They can be set up by a relative or, commonly, by the community pharmacist. If the patient already uses one of these and an additional prescription is needed, then liaison with the pharmacist or carer is necessary to ensure correct administration.

Further advice on prescribing in older people is given in the British National Formulary.[6]

CONCLUSION

Older people in general are frequent users of dental care and the frail elderly patient with disabilities and multiple medical problems provides a particular challenge. The patient's general medical practitioner and their relatives or carers are an essential source of information and help in the delivery of dental treatment.

1. Department of Health. National service framework for older people. London: Department of Health, 2001. http://www.dh.gov.uk/en/Publicationsandstatistics/Publications/PublicationsPolicyAndGuidance/DH_4003066.
2. Janzen P R M, Christys A, Vucevic M. Patient-controlled sedation using propofol in elderly patients in day-case cataract surgery. *Br J Anaesth* 1999; **82:** 635–636.
3. Arias E. United States life tables, 2000. Natl *Vital Stat Rep* 2002; **51:** 1–38.
4. Daublander M, Muller R, Lipp M D W. The incidence of complications associated with local anesthesia in dentistry. *Anesth Prog* 1997; **44:** 132–141.
5. Nordenram A, Danielsson K. Local anaesthesia in elderly patients. An experimental study of oral infiltration anaesthesia. *Swed Dent J* 1990; **14:** 19–24.
6. British national formulary 55. London: BMJ Publishing Group/Pharmaceutical Press, 2009. www.bnf.org.
7. Colquhoun M C, Daly M, Stewart P, Beeley L. Interaction between warfarin and miconazole oral gel. *Lancet* 1987; **1(8534):** 695–696.

Chapter 12
Metabolic disorders

M. Greenwood and J. G. Meechan

IN BRIEF

- Metabolic disorders, or drugs which affect metabolism, are commonly seen in dental patients.
- There will often be no physical signs in the patient with metabolic problems.
- A thorough history is particularly important and a thorough family history will often uncover important findings.
- Knowledge of metabolic disorders will highlight patients who need special precautions to facilitate safe treatment.

It is important for dental practitioners to have a basic knowledge of the more common metabolic disorders as some may impact on the practice of dentistry. Many of these disorders do not have overt clinical signs. Taking a thorough medical history and where necessary, liaising with the patient's physician, is particularly important.

INTRODUCTION

Knowledge of metabolic disorders is essential for the safe management of dental patients. This chapter considers conditions that impact on the practice of dentistry.

POINTS IN THE HISTORY

Several points in the history may reveal an underlying metabolic disorder (*Table 1*).

Hypercholesterolaemia

Hypercholesterolaemia is a condition which has received significant attention in recent years. It has little significance for the provision of local anaesthesia but the possibility

of ischaemic heart disease should be remembered. Low density lipoproteins (LDL) are associated with a higher risk of coronary heart disease. They are formed from intermediate density lipoproteins in the liver and contain a core of cholesterol. They bind to LDL receptors and are taken up by cells. This is particularly so when there is inhibition of 3-hydroxy-3-methylglutaryl coenzyme A reductase (HMG CoA reductase), which raises cellular cholesterol. On the other hand, high density lipoproteins (HDL) are associated with a reduced risk of coronary heart disease. They carry cholesterol back to the liver from intercellular tissue.

Porphyrias

Porphyrias are rare disorders but potentially impact on dental treatment. They arise principally as the result of errors in haem metabolism causing accumulation of porphyrins, which are intermediate compounds in haemoglobin synthesis. Two main groups are recognised. These are the liver (hepatic) porphyrias and the red blood cell (erythropoietic) porphyrias. Patients with porphyrias may remain asymptomatic, but acute illness or drugs may precipitate an attack.

Variegate porphyria is the commonest form and is found mainly in people of Afrikaans descent. **Acute intermittent porphyria** affects all populations but is seen

Table 1 Points in the history in patients with metabolic disorders
Hypercholesterolaemia
Porphyria (or subtypes)
Malignant hyperpyrexia
Neuroleptic malignant syndrome
G6PD deficiency
Suxamethonium apnoea
Haemochromatosis
Amyloidosis
Abnormalities of carbohydrate metabolism

less frequently. A further form, **hereditary coproporphyria** is also recognised.

Between attacks a patient with porphyria may appear normal although they may have photosensitive skin resulting in rashes. An acute attack may result in neuropsychiatric symptoms. Porphyria that becomes acute as a result of drugs may cause cardiovascular symptoms such as hypertension and tachycardia. Gastrointestinal symptoms may also occur. Some of the drugs that dentists prescribe can induce an acute attack of porphyria. Details of these are given later.

Malignant hyperpyrexia

Malignant hyperpyrexia (MH) is a rare but potentially fatal condition. It is inherited and presents as a rapid temperature rise if the patient is subjected to general anaesthesia or other medications. The family history may elicit a history of MH. Two forms are recognised: firstly, an autosomal dominant type where patients are normal between attacks, and secondly, a recessive form that affects boys with muscle disorders, for example myotonic dystrophy.

The most common trigger of MH is a combination of halothane[1] (an anaesthetic agent) and muscle relaxants including suxamethonium.[2] The rising temperature is accompanied by tachycardia or arrhythmias and hypotension. Management involves removing the precipitating cause, cooling and hyperventilating the patient to correct any respiratory acidosis and the use of dantrolene.

Neuroleptic malignant syndrome

Neuroleptic malignant syndrome (NMS) is rare but again potentially fatal. It is induced by the administration of certain drugs, but none commonly used in dentistry. It is recognised clinically by disturbance in the patient's mental state, autonomic function and temperature regulation.

Glucose-6-phosphate dehydrogenase deficiency

Patients may give a history of known glucose–6-phosphate dehydrogenase (G6PD) deficiency. This is the most common enzyme deficiency seen mainly in people of Mediterranean, African, Asian or Middle Eastern descent. Glucose can be metabolised via the glycolytic or the hexose monophosphate shunt pathways (*Fig. 1*). G6PD is involved in the latter. A derivative of the hexose monophosphate shunt is NADPH, which is involved in removing dangerous oxidative metabolites. If the activity of G6PD is low, **methaemoglobinaemia** (oxidised haemoglobin molecule) results and when red cells are exposed to oxidising agents, sometimes present in drugs, haemolysis results. Diagnosis is confirmed by measuring levels of the enzyme. The haemolysis is usually self-limiting but occasionally splenectomy is required .

Suxamethonium apnoea

Sensitivity to suxamethonium or scoline ('scoline apnoea') is sometimes seen and patients are often aware of its existence in the family. It is inherited as an autosomal recessive trait. Suxamethonium is a muscle relaxant that acts as a depolarising neuromuscular blocker. It behaves in a similar way to acetylcholine at the neuromuscular junction. Its action is usually brief since it is quickly destroyed by plasma cholinesterase. Around 1 in 2,000 of the population has a defect in plasma cholinesterase. This makes such people abnormally sensitive when suxamethonium is administered, resulting in persistent muscle paralysis. This means that the patients are unable to breathe for themselves (apnoea). It is postulated that the disorder may be a form of hypersensitivity reaction.

Haemochromatosis

Patients may give a history of haemochromatosis. This is a disorder of iron metabolism resulting in too much iron being absorbed from the intestine, which causes high serum ferritin levels. Deposition of iron occurs in the liver, joints, skin, adrenal glands and various other organs including the heart. The iron is deposited as haemosiderin. This is more problematic in males than females due to menstrual blood loss. The haemosiderin deposits provoke a fibrotic reaction that can produce disorders wherever the deposits are found, resulting in disorders such as cirrhosis, adrenocortical insufficiency, cardiomyopathy, skin pigmentation and diabetes (so-called 'bronze' diabetes). The condition is treated by blood letting to reduce the iron load and sometimes medically using the chelating agent desferrioxamine.

Amyloidosis

Amyloidosis (*Fig. 2*) is a disorder characterised by the deposition of eosinophilic hyaline protein in the tissues. It is really a manifestation of disease processes. It can affect the functions of the heart, gastrointestinal tract, spleen, kidney, liver and

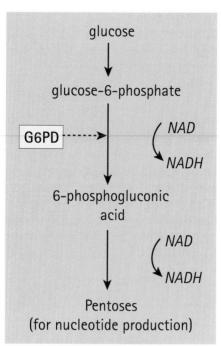

Fig. 1 The role of glucose-6-phosphate dehydrogenase (G6PD) in the hexose monophosphate shunt pathway

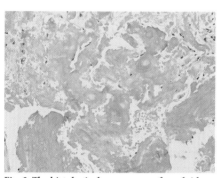

Fig. 2 The histological appearance of amyloid stained with Congo Red

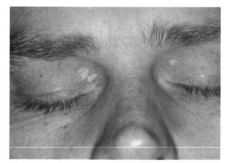

Fig. 3 Xanthelasmas in the eyelids

adrenals when it is deposited there. There may also be a bleeding tendency due to a Factor X defect.

Abnormalities of carbohydrate metabolism

Defects in carbohydrate metabolism are uncommon but may be seen in dental patients. The two main conditions are glycogen storage diseases and defects in fructose metabolism. In the glycogen storage disorders there is accumulation of the polysaccharide as a result of inherited defects in the enzymes that metabolise it. This causes hypoglycaemia. The glycogen accumulates preferentially in liver and muscle resulting in an enlarged liver, muscle pain and weakness (including the respiratory muscles). Heart failure may also supervene. One subdivision of glycogen storage disease produces a bleeding tendency.

EXAMINATION OF THE DENTAL PATIENT WITH A METABOLIC DISORDER

There is often little to be seen in patients with metabolic disorders that would facilitate diagnosis of their condition. Some observations which may give a clue to an underlying metabolic condition are discussed below.

Xanthomas are yellowish plaques that may be apparent on the skin. These are termed xanthelasmas when on the eyelids (*Fig. 3*). They are seen in familial hyperlipidaemia and are associated with accelerated atherosclerosis and coronary heart disease.

In haemochromatosis, the skin may take on a bronze hue. Patients with porphyria may be subject to photosensitive skin rashes.

Amyloidosis may only be diagnosed formally by biopsy. It can present with an intraoral lesion, for example deposition in the tongue may lead to enlargement or localised swelling. The gingivae may also be affected. Bullae and petechiae may be seen intra-orally.

DENTAL MANAGEMENT OF PATIENTS WITH METABOLIC DISORDERS

It should be remembered in the patient with hypercholesterolaemia that there is an increased risk of ischaemic heart disease. This heightens the risks of general anaesthesia. Conscious sedation is a suitable alternative but local anaesthesia is the preferred method.

The safest management of a patient with porphyria is care with drug prescription. This is discussed below. It should be borne in mind, however,

that data in this area are still incomplete. Thus the prescription of drugs in this group of patients should be carried out with this in mind.

Some drugs should be avoided in cases with G6PD deficiency for fear of producing haemolysis. The only drugs that may be used in the practice of dentistry that fall into this category are the sulphonamide antibacterial drugs.

In patients with malignant hyperpyrexia (MH), it is important to treat infections promptly and aggressively as they are known to be potential precipitants of an attack. It is safe to give local anaesthetics. The response to adrenaline (epinephrine) may be similar to the early signs of an MH reaction and this should be remembered. Such signs include tachycardia, rising blood pressure and rapid breathing. Adrenaline also potentiates the release of calcium in muscle cells, which theoretically would enhance MH; because of this dose limitation is important. The use of sedation in patients with MH is discussed below.

In patients with suxamethonium sensitivity, a careful history will usually uncover this; however some patients may be unaware of the condition. The use of local anaesthetics in such cases is discussed below.

Drugs that may be used in the practice of dentistry that are considered unsafe in patients with porphyria include tricyclic and monoamine anti-depressants, sulphonamides, anticonvulsant medications such as carbamazepine and phenytoin, diazepam, chloral hydrate and triclofos, clindamycin, doxycycline, erythromycin, ketoconazole, metronidazole, miconazole and oxytetracycline.

Factors affecting dental treatment under local anaesthesia, sedation, general anaesthesia and management in dental practice

The first step is to obtain a full history, which will alert the practitioner to the patient suffering from a metabolic disorder. Many patients will have no overt clinical signs.

The patient with hypercholesterolaemia is best treated under local anaesthesia, but conscious sedation is a suitable mode of treatment. The risk of ischaemic heart disease should be remembered with general anaesthesia.

In the patient with porphyria, consideration needs to be given in the use of local anaesthesia as sodium metabisulphite, which is contained in some local anaesthetic preparations to prevent the oxidation of adrenaline, can precipitate an attack.[3] Lidocaine and prilocaine are considered safe when administered for local anaesthesia.

Local anaesthesia is considered safe in patients who give a history of malignant hyperpyrexia.[4] As stated earlier, however, adrenaline can produce similar signs to the early stages of MH and this should be remembered. It is therefore wise to limit the dose of adrenaline in these patients. Adrenaline should not be used as a topical agent to manage gingival bleeding in such patients.

Benzodiazepines are not considered to be triggers of MH and conscious sedation using inhalation sedation is usually safe.[4] MH has, however, been reported after inhalation of nitrous oxide[5] but this is very rare.

In patients with G6PD deficiency, local anaesthesia may induce methaemoglobinaemia in high doses. The most likely candidates are prilocaine and the topical agent benzocaine.[6] Inhalation sedation is usually safe. General anaesthesia should be given in a hospital environment. The use of large doses of aspirin and the sulphonamide antibacterial drugs may precipitate haemolysis in patients with G6PD deficiency and should be avoided.

Patients with suxamethonium sensitivity may metabolise local anaesthetics differently from normal. As mentioned above this condition results from defects in plasma esterases. All of the injectable local anaesthetics used in modern dental practice are amides, unlike the earlier ester procaine. Nevertheless one of the amides, articaine, is initially metabolised in plasma by esterases[7] so the use of this drug in patients with suxamethonium sensitivity may increase the toxicity of the anaesthetic. If a patient's history reveals sensitivity to suxamethonium they can be safely treated under general anaesthetic with avoidance of this muscle relaxant.

Haemochromatosis affects dental management in many ways, although local anaesthesia is usually safe. The possibility of cirrhosis, cardiomyopathy, diabetes and adrenocortical insufficiency should be borne in mind in these patients. Providing that liver function is adequate, conscious sedation is usually safe.

Local anaesthesia and conscious sedation can safely be given in patients with amyloidosis in most cases. It should be remembered, however, that amyloid can affect diverse organ systems. If the heart, adrenal glands or kidneys are involved or a bleeding tendency has developed, this will affect function and/or haemostasis.

Methaemoglobinaemia is a conversion of iron in haemoglobin from the ferrous to the ferric form. This latter configuration of iron does not allow such good availability of oxygen to the tissues which can result in cyanosis. Methaemoglobinaemia is a side effect of injecting large doses of some local anaesthetics, especially prilocaine[8] and articaine. Thus if using these drugs dose limitations should be employed or an alternative local anaesthetic should be used in the anaemic patient.

Effects of drugs used in patients with metabolic disorders on dental management

Some of the lipid-regulating drugs can increase bleeding after surgery. The anion-exchange resins colestyramine and colestipol may interfere with the absorption of vitamin K leading to hypoprothrombinaemia. Ezetimibe, which interferes with the absorption of cholesterol, may rarely cause a reduction in platelet numbers. The fibrates, such as bezafibrate, may also cause a thrombocytopaenia as well as reducing white cell numbers and causing anaemia.

Statins such as atorvastatin can also produce a thrombocytopaenia. Thrombocytopaenia with a platelet count of less than 50×10^9/litre precludes elective oral surgery; when levels are less than 100×10^9/litre, tooth sockets should be packed with a haemostatic agent and sutured. Omega-3-acid ethyl esters can occasionally produce taste disturbance.

A number of drugs may be prescribed in the management of amyloidosis. The use of cytotoxic drugs and corticosteroids such as dexamethasone can lead to opportunistic oral infections, delayed healing and poor haemostasis. Colchicine, which is sometimes used in symptomatic treatment, can produce stomatitis and glossitis.

Drug interactions with drugs used in dentistry

One of the unwanted effects of statins is myopathy. The incidence of this is increased when statins are administered concurrently with other drugs, some of which may be prescribed to treat orofacial conditions. The important drugs in this regard are the antibacterial erythromycin and the azole antifungals. Erythromycin, itraconazole, ketoconazole and miconazole should not be prescribed to patients receiving simvastatin. Similarly, itraconazole should be avoided in patients taking atorvastatin. The toxicity of colchicine is increased during concurrent therapy with erythromycin.

CONCLUSIONS

Metabolic disorders can impact on dental treatment in diverse ways. A thorough history and a high index of suspicion are essential for safe patient management.

1. Fukami M C, Ganzberg S I. A case report of malignant hyperthermia in a dental clinic operating room. *Anesth Prog* 2005; **52:** 24–28.
2. Monaghan A, Hindle I. Malignant hyperpyrexia in oral surgery – case report and literature review. *Br J Oral Maxillofac Surg* 1994; **32:** 190–193.
3. Brown G J, Welbury R R. Porphyria in dental practice. *Br Dent J* 2002; **193:** 145–146.
4. Malignant Hyperthermia Association of the United States. Malignant hyperthermia. A concern in dentistry and oral and maxillofacial surgery. Sherburne, NY: MHAUS, 2002. http://www.mhaus.org/index.cfm/fuseaction/OnlineBrochures.Display/BrochurePK/ABD1DA74-4433-48F3-A4C7902B67F6FCFB.cfm.
5. Ellis F R, Clarke I M C, Appleyard T N, Dinsdale R C W. Malignant hyperthermia induced by nitrous oxide and treated with dexamethasone. *Br Med J* 1974; **4:** 270–271.
6. Coleman M D, Coleman N A. Drug-induced methaemoglobinaemia. Treatment issues. *Drug Saf* 1996; **14:** 394–405.
7. Oertel R, Rahn R, Kirch W. Clinical pharmacokinetics of articaine. *Clin Pharmacokinet* 1997; **33:** 417–245.
8. Adams V, Marley J, McCarroll C. Prilocaine induced methaemoglobinaemia in a medically compromised patient. Was this an inevitable consequence of the dose administered? *Br Dent J* 2007; **203:** 585–587.

Chapter 13
Skin disorders part A

M. Greenwood, J. G. Meechan, R. I. Macleod and M. Rudralingam

IN BRIEF

- A dentist should have a sound knowledge of skin disorders, particularly those which have oral manifestations.
- History and examination (lesion recognition) is important.
- Some of the treatments for skin disorders, particularly steroid treatment, may impact on dental treatment and should be borne in mind.

Skin disorders are potentially important to dentists in diverse ways. The skin disease itself might have oral manifestations, and drugs used to treat skin disorders may impact on dental management. This first chapter considering skin disorders examines points to look out for in the history and considers specific groups of conditions. Further conditions will be discussed in chapter 14.

INTRODUCTION

The skin is subject to a number of disorders that can arise as a result of external insults such as trauma and infection, internal factors due to systemic disease, and disorders specific to the skin itself. Skin disorders can be congenital, developmental or acquired.

As areas of the skin such as the hands and face are visible, they can be easily examined in the clothed patient. Some skin conditions may present with oral manifestations that can occur either simultaneously or precede the main dermatological features.

This consideration of dermatology is divided into two chapters. The first concentrates on general principles. In addition, the conditions summarised in the first part of *Table 1* are considered. Further disorders (the second part of *Table 1*) will be discussed in chapter 14.

Dermatology is a descriptive subject with an extensive range and variety of conditions that often appear clinically very similar and can only be differentiated histologically. *Table 2* gives some commonly used terms and definitions of skin conditions.

Table 1 Broad categories that can be applied to skin disorders

- Lumps and bumps
- Malignant conditions
- Rashes
- Collagen vascular diseases
- Blistering disorders*
- Skin infections*
- Disorders of hair*
- Disorders of pigmentation.*

*Considered in chapter 14

Table 2 Examination and description of a skin rash

Macule	An area of discolouration. May be more red or paler than the surrounding skin, or may be a different colour, eg blue
Papule	A small raised area. A maculopapular rash is both raised and discoloured
Nodule	A firm papule (more than 0.5 cm diameter)
Vesicle	A small blister (less than 0.5 cm diameter)
Bulla	A large blister (more than 0.5 cm diameter)
Pustule	A papule that contains pus
Erythema	Redness due to increased perfusion of the skin
Scale	A flake of easily detached keratin
Crust	An accumulation of dried exudate
Atrophy	Thinning of skin, often with loss of skin markings and increased translucency
Sclerosis	An induration of the dermis, usually due to increased collagen
Excoriation	A scratch mark
Ulcer	A breach in the epidermis, which may range from a small superficial erosion to a massive defect of skin and underlying tissue

POINTS IN THE HISTORY

Patients with skin conditions present in a variety of ways. Such presentations can include the appearance (or change in appearance) of a lesion, a rash or an itch – the latter can vary from being a minor nuisance to a debilitating problem interfering with sleep. In addition, itching usually leads to scratching with resultant damage to the skin, pain, secondary infection and scarring. In some instances the skin disorder may be asymptomatic and the patient only presents after it is pointed out to them.

A thorough history is essential to making a diagnosis; this includes relevant past medical history and systemic enquiry. For skin conditions, the history should include specific questions about onset, any change in appearance over time, exacerbating and relieving factors and possible causative factors such as contact with potential infection or allergens; details about occupation and exposure to ultraviolet light (sunlight or sun-beds - *Table 3*) are also important.

As many skin conditions, such as atopic eczema and psoriasis, have a genetic element, a family history should be included. When considering rashes, their spread and distribution over the body is an important feature, as many have a characteristic pattern. When oral mucosa is involved, tactful questioning about lesions of the genital and conjunctival mucosa should be made.

CATEGORISATION OF SKIN DISORDERS

A categorisation of skin disorders is given in *Table 1*, and these are discussed below and continued in chapter 14.

1. Lumps and bumps

Basal cell papilloma (seborrhoeic wart) is a pigmented lesion which commonly occurs in the elderly (*Fig 1*). It has a characteristic warty surface, often with a greasy appearance. It is unrelated to the more aggressive basal cell carcinoma and treatment is usually for cosmetic purposes using either surgical removal or cryotherapy.

Table 3 Points in the history of a patient with a skin disorder
• Onset
• Change in appearance over time
• Exacerbating or relieving factors
• Possible causative factors:
○ Infections
○ Allergen contact
○ Exposure to ultraviolet light (sunshine or sun beds)
• If a rash, is it itchy?
• Past medical history
• Systemic enquiry
• Family history.

Keratoacanthoma is a rapidly growing lesion which develops into a dome shaped lump with a central keratin filled crater (*Fig. 2*). The lesion can resemble a squamous cell carcinoma but may resolve spontaneously.

Pyogenic granuloma usually presents as a rapidly developing red lump that bleeds readily when touched (*Fig. 3*). In many cases there is a history of trauma to the area before the appearance of the lump and it actually represents excess production of granulation tissue. These lesions are usually either surgically removed or treated with cryotherapy.

Epidermoid cyst is a common cystic lesion of the scalp, filled with a cheesy keratinous material. These lesions are commonly called sebaceous cysts although this term is a misnomer. The usual treatment is surgical removal.

2. Vascular anomalies

There are a number of vascular anomalies that can affect the skin and all can be identified as having a vascular nature by blanching on pressure. **Campbell de Morgan** spots are small capillary haemangiomas that occur on the trunk with increasing age and are of no significance. They should not, however, be confused with **hereditary haemorrhagic telangiectasia (HHT)**, which as the name implies has a genetic factor and can present with numerous red 'spots' around the lips as well as in other areas. HHT can lead to extensive bleeding from the nasal passages and bowel leading to iron deficiency anaemia. As a result, individual lesions may need to

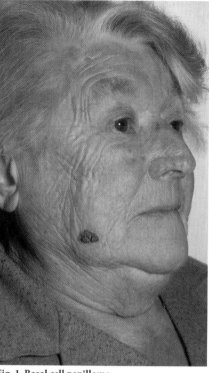
Fig. 1 Basal cell papilloma

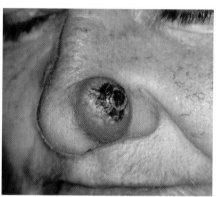
Fig. 2 Keratoacanthoma

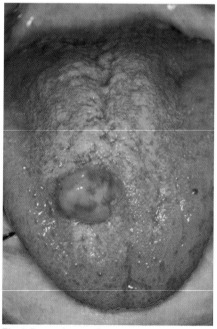
Fig. 3 Pyogenic granuloma

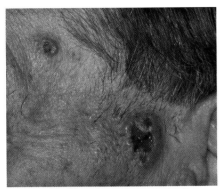

Fig. 4 Basal cell carcinoma ('rodent ulcer')

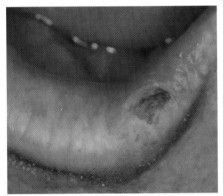

Fig. 5 Squamous cell cancer of lower lip

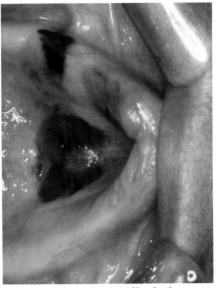

Fig. 6 Malignant melanoma of hard palate

Table 4 Factors suggestive of possible malignancy in a pigmented lesion
• Progressive enlargement • Colour change • Spread of pigment beyond the edges of the lesion • Bleeding, itching or inflammation.

be cauterised.

'Port-wine stain' is a more extensive capillary haemangioma that is present at birth and can cause a considerable cosmetic problem. They can be treated by laser,[1] however some resort to cosmetic camouflage. Lesions on the face are occasionally associated with vascular malformations in the brain and resultant epilepsy. It is worth considering that lesions affecting the mandible or maxilla may extend into the adjacent bone and could pose a problem with dental extractions in the area. In such cases a pre-operative radiograph should be taken and if involvement is shown, referral for angiography should be arranged.

Strawberry naevus is a term used to describe a vascular malformation that presents in infancy as a raised red lump. Such lesions initially appear to enlarge but eventually regress and consequently treatment should, if possible, be deferred until adolescence.

3. Malignant conditions

The most important factor predisposing to malignancy of the skin is ultraviolet radiation, and most cutaneous malignancy occurs on parts of the body exposed to light. As well as producing damage to genes, ultraviolet light may cause immunosuppression and this may be implicated in its role in carcinogenesis.[2] Other causes of skin cancer include X-rays, chemicals (eg arsenic and benzpyrene) and genetic factors. Lesions in this group include basal cell carcinoma and squamous cell carcinoma.

Basal cell carcinoma ('rodent ulcer') characteristically appears as a pearly papule that enlarges slowly and then ulcerates to form an ulcer with a rolled edge (*Fig. 4*). Although these lesions do not metastasise, they are locally aggressive and destructive and require prompt referral. Treatment is usually surgical excision, although some lesions can be treated with radiotherapy.

Squamous cell carcinoma (SCC) often arises on skin that shows evidence of sun induced degenerative changes (eg solar elastosis or keratosis). The lesion may present as an indurated lump or an ulcer with a firm base (*Fig. 5*). Lesions require surgical excision and careful follow up. Affected patients need advice on limiting future exposure to ultraviolet light and need to be aware of changes in other areas of pre-existing solar damaged skin. **Bowen's disease** is a patch of non-invasive squamous cell carcinoma. It may mimic psoriasis and has a relatively good prognosis.

Melanotic lesions of the skin are common and represent collections of melanocytes within the epidermis, dermis or sub-dermal tissues. A variety of descriptive terms are used depending on the clinical appearance and histological distribution of the melanocytes, but all are commonly referred to as 'moles'. **Melanocytic naevus** (intradermal naevus) is due to melanocytes congregating in the dermis. They may develop at any time, but commonly enlarge during puberty or pregnancy. They may be variably pigmented, flat or raised, hairy or hairless. They are essentially a cosmetic defect and rarely become malignant.

Malignant melanoma originates from melanocytes and may arise in a pre-existing mole or in otherwise normal skin or oral mucosa (*Fig. 6*). Factors that raise suspicion of malignant change in a pre-existing pigmented lesion include progressive enlargement, colour change, spread of pigment beyond the edge of the lesion, bleeding, itching or inflammation (*Table 4*). Any such changes require urgent referral as malignant melanomas have a propensity to metastasise widely at a relatively early stage. Treatment is usually surgical excision with a wide margin and careful follow up.

4. Rashes

Rashes are common. Most have a short duration and accompany viral infections, especially in childhood. A few are the main manifestation of the illness, such as in chickenpox, rubella (German measles) or measles. In this section the non-infectious causes of rashes are considered.

Eczema is a distinctive inflammation of the skin in which the prickle cells of the epidermis become separated from each other by oedema fluid. Eczema is characterised by severe itching and erythema, with a variable degree of papule formation, vesiculation, scaling and weeping.

Eczema can be divided into two main types: exogenous, due to an external cause, and endogenous, due to either an internal or unknown cause.

Exogenous eczema includes:
- Primary irritant eczema – arises as a result of irritants such as caustics, mineral oils and detergents. Occupational hand eczema is often due to regular contact with these chemicals
- Allergic contact dermatitis is due to a Type IV (delayed) hypersensitivity reaction and may develop to a variety of substances such as nickel, rubber and dyes (discussed further in chapter 14).

Endogenous eczema usually begins in infancy and tends to clear during childhood. Severe cases can be life-long. In many instances there is a family history and the condition may be associated with hay fever, urticaria and asthma ('atopic' patients). It is an interesting observation that in such patients when their eczema is bad, their asthma improves and *vice versa*.

Most affected individuals can control their skin condition with topical emollients and intermittent topical steroids and only in a few cases are systemic steroids required. Courses are usually kept for as brief a time as possible. In addition to conventional therapy a number of atopic patients could be using various complementary therapies, which may be self-prescribed. It is known that some of these, in particular herbal remedies, can interfere with medication such as antibiotics and it is worth checking what the patient is using before issuing a prescription.

Seborrhoeic dermatitis is an ill-defined type of eczema, classically causing dandruff, scaly eyebrows, redness of the naso-labial folds and patches of red rash over the sternum and in the body folds. Some patients have a greasy skin, but the term 'seborrhoeic' is probably a misnomer. Although the exact cause of this condition is unknown, the role of *Pityrosporum* yeasts has been recently emphasised. The condition is usually controlled with topical steroids, tar-based products and antifungal medication.

Varicose eczema affects the lower leg and is due to venous stasis. The affected skin often becomes irritable and pigmented. The affected area can readily ulcerate following often mild trauma. Management is usually symptomatic.

Psoriasis is a common inflammatory skin disease with well-demarcated patches of red skin covered with thick white scales (*Fig . 7*). The most commonly affected areas are the extensor surfaces, knees, elbows and base of spine. There are a number of recognised subtypes but apart from the scalp, the face is rarely affected. The exact cause of psoriasis remains unknown, although in a number of cases there is a strong family history.

The basic abnormality in psoriasis appears to be an increased rate of epidermal regeneration of the affected skin. Some patients develop an associated arthritis (psoriatic arthropathy) and pitting of the finger nails. Psoriasis can range from being a minor nuisance to a life-threatening incapacity. There are numerous therapies advocated for psoriasis, which depend on the severity of the condition but include topical coal tar preparations, steroids, ultraviolet radiation and systemic treatments such as retinoids (vitamin A analogues).

Acne vulgaris is a common disease of adolescence and is characterised by greasy skin (seborrhoea), blackheads (comedones), papules and pustules. In addition, there may be deep-seated cysts which tend to leave pitted scars. Lesions start on the face and may spread to the shoulders, back and chest. The condition starts around puberty, when sebaceous glands become active due to androgenic stimulation. Colonisation with anaerobic diphtheroids follows, which break down the sebum to free fatty acids causing comedone formation. The exact cause

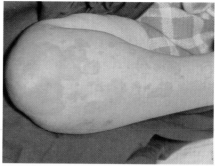
Fig. 7 Psoriasis

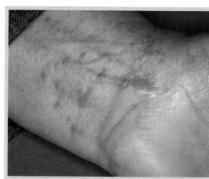

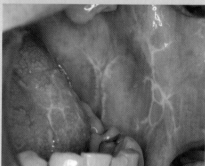
Fig. 8 The skin and oral lesions of lichen planus

of the subsequent inflammation is unknown. Antibiotics such as tetracycline decrease the bacterial count and suppress inflammation.

Acne rosacea is a skin disorder of the middle aged and elderly characterised by redness, papules and pustules of the face, a tendency to facial flushing and telangiectasia. The condition is exacerbated by sunlight and heat and can be distinguished from acne vulgaris by the absence of comedones and scarring. The exact cause of the condition is unknown and treatment is similar as for acne vulgaris.

Lichen planus is a disorder of unknown aetiology. It is characterised by flat topped, violaceous papules which are extremely itchy (*Fig. 8*). The most common sites affected are the flexor surfaces of the wrists, the shins and midriff; the face is rarely involved. The oral mucosa is frequently affected with white streaks, often with a reticulate pattern and is predominantly found on the buccal mucosa and lateral margins of the tongue (*Fig. 8*) although a number of different clinical features may be present.[3] The oral lesions may become erosive and painful and chronic cases have a slightly increased risk of malignant transformation.

The natural history of lichen planus is for gradual resolution over 18 months to two years leaving residual pigmented macules. However, oral involvement can take much longer to resolve and can last for years. Treatment depends on severity and usually involves topical steroids[4] with only the more severe cases requiring systemic treatment. More intractable disease can respond to specific immunomodulating drugs such as ciclosporin or tacrolimus.

Urticaria is a blotchy rash, characterised by wheals, erythema and itching. It usually develops rapidly, fading within 24 hours. The condition is a result of histamine release from mast cells increasing capillary permeability and giving a red axon flare. It is often due to a Type I hypersensitivity reaction to a specific food (for example, shellfish), food additives or drugs. In many cases no specific trigger is found and treatment is symptomatic with either avoidance of the trigger substance or antihistamines.

Angio-oedema is a similar condition to urticaria but the increased capillary permeability occurs at a deeper level, with swelling of the subcutaneous tissues. It most commonly affects the eyelids and lips. Rarely, it may cause respiratory obstruction due to laryngeal oedema in which case the condition becomes a medical emergency requiring the immediate use of intramuscular adrenaline, otherwise the condition is managed in the same way as urticaria.

It should be remembered that cases due to a Type I hypersensitivity can have an exaggerated response on subsequent contact with the provoking allergen and can develop a potentially fatal anaphylaxis. In view of such a possibility affected patients are advised to carry an emergency supply of adrenaline for self-administration in an 'EpiPen'®.

A similar presentation to angio-oedema can arise due a genetic disorder in which a component of the control of the complement cascade is missing (C1 esterase inhibitor) with the result that minor trauma, including possible tissue handling during dental treatment, can provoke an inflammatory response with localised oedematous swelling. This condition is usually much less severe than its hypersensitivity counterpart and episodes settle without the need for intervention.

5. Collagen vascular diseases

Lupus erythematosus (LE) is an autoimmune disorder in which antibodies are directed against the skin. It can present in two forms, discoid LE and systemic LE.

Discoid LE (DLE) is a disease confined to the skin, although antinuclear factor may be present in the blood. The rash is characterised by disc shaped areas of redness with scaling and atrophy and mainly affects the sun-exposed areas of the skin, including the face. The condition is exacerbated by sunlight and consequently is worse during the summer months. About 5% of affected patients progress to the systemic form.

In **systemic LE (SLE)** the rash tends to be nonspecific, though classically patients develop a 'butterfly' distribution over the cheeks and bridge of nose, reflecting the photosensitive nature of the condition. The systemic changes are variable but may include pyrexia, malaise, arthralgia, pleurisy, pericarditis, renal failure and neuropsychiatric involvement. Both DLE and SLE require specialist treatment. Such treatment often involves protracted courses of systemic steroids and steroid sparing immunomodulating medication such as methotrexate.

DLE and SLE can produce oral lesions which vary from non-specific mucosal ulceration to lesions with a lichenoid appearance. There is also an association between SLE and the development of dry eyes and dry mouth (Sjögren's syndrome) with oral consequences such as increased rate of dental caries, periodontal disease and secondary Candidal infection.

Systemic sclerosis is a chronic and ultimately fatal condition often presenting with Raynaud's phenomenon (painful vascular spasm of the extremities, usually fingers, triggered by cold) some years before an insidious induration of the skin develops. Facial changes are pathognomic and include immobile 'bound down' skin, small mouth with radial furrows and loss of bulk in the nasal alae – the result giving a taught, smooth skinned appearance. More systemic (and potentially fatal) involvement includes pulmonary fibrosis, loss of oesophageal peristalsis, renal failure and in the latter stages, progressive digital ischaemia with gangrene, ulceration and loss of digits.

Dermatomyositis is an autoimmune inflammatory disorder affecting skin and muscle. The rash is non-specific, but a violaceous rash of the eyelids and red plaques over the knuckles suggest the diagnosis. A progressive proximal myopathy causes difficulty in climbing steps and eventually limits mobility. The disorder is associated with internal malignancy in 50% of middle-aged patients. A similar condition seen in children does not have the same association with malignancy.

Polyarteritis nodosa is an autoimmune disorder resulting in a necrotising vasculitis occurring in medium sized arteries. Any organ may be affected but the skin involvement includes a blotchy reticulate cyanosis (livedo reticularis), haemorrhagic blisters and irregular punched-out ulcers. There are many milder forms of vasculitis affecting smaller vessels only, with lesions confined to the skin. Some of these disorders are a result of circulating immune complexes.

CONCLUSIONS

There are several skin conditions which can be encountered by dental practitioners. Some may be incidental findings but others may be part of the oral condition. A thorough history and examination is important in every case.

On occasion, treatments being received for the skin condition may have a direct impact on dental management. This, together with further skin conditions will be considered in chapter 14.

1. Stier M F, Glick S A, Hirsch R J. Laser treatment of pediatric vascular lesions: Port wine stains and haemangiomas. *J Am Acad Dermatol* 2008; **58:** 261–285.
2. Welsh M M, Karagas M R, Applebaum K M, Spencer S K, Perry A E, Nelson H H. A role for ultraviolet radiation immunosuppression in non-melanoma skin cancer as evidenced by gene-environment interactions. *Carcinogenesis* 2008; **29:** 1950–1954.
3. McCartan B E, Healy C M. The reported prevalence of oral lichen planus: a review and critique. *J Oral Pathol Med* 2008; **37:** 447–453.
4. Thongprasom K, Dhanuthai K. Steroids in the treatment of lichen planus: a review. *J Oral Sci* 2008; **50:** 377–385.

Chapter 14
Skin disorders part B

M. Greenwood, J. G. Meechan, R. I. Macleod and M. Rudralingam

IN BRIEF

- Skin disorders are common and are likely to be encountered by dental practitioners.
- History and examination (lesion recognition) is important.
- The skin disorder may have oral manifestations.
- Some treatments for skin disorders may impact on dental management. The more important areas where treatments may affect dental management are discussed in this chapter.

Skin disorders are potentially important to dentists in diverse ways. The skin disease itself might have oral manifestations, and drugs used to treat skin disorders may impact on dental management. This chapter on skin disorders continues with a consideration of those disorders, and aspects of their treatment, which could have relevance to dental practitioners.

INTRODUCTION

In chapter 13 general aspects of the history and examination of a patient with a skin lesion were discussed. Several specific conditions were highlighted. This chapter continues with a consideration of further skin conditions and aspects of management as they impact on dental treatment. The skin conditions covered in this paper are summarised in *Table 1*.

1. BLISTERING DISORDERS

Blistering disorders may be classified according to where the split in the skin leading to the blisters occurs.

Intra-epidermal blisters tend to have a thin roof and rupture easily whereas those occurring sub-epidermally rupture less readily and present with tense, dome shaped blisters.

There are a number of subtypes of **pemphigus,**[1] all of which are autoimmune with the autoantibodies (usually IgG) directed against the 'cement' of the prickle cell layer of the epidermis with resultant breakdown and blister formation in this region. Patients, most frequently middle-aged women, present with widespread flaccid blisters of the skin but often involving the mucous membranes of the mouth, conjunctiva, nose, vagina and rectum. In roughly 50% of patients the condition may first manifest as an oral problem. Pemphigus, if untreated, is fatal and warrants vigorous and life-long immunosuppressive treatment.

Pemphigoid is also an autoimmune disorder that usually occurs in the older patient and tends to be a much milder condition than pemphigus. The autoantibodies, usually IgG, are directed towards the basement membrane zone resulting in sub-epidermal blister formation. It tends to spare the mucous membranes but a variant, **mucous membrane pemphigoid,**[2] predominantly involves the oral and conjunctival mucosa. The latter is of significance because, if not treated, it can lead to conjunctival scarring and blindness. Pemphigoid is usually treated symptomatically with topical steroids and only in severe cases is

Table 1 A summary of the conditions discussed in this chapter
Blistering disorders
Skin infections
Disorders of hair
Disorders of pigmentation
Miscellaneous conditions

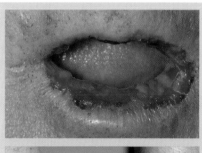
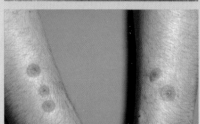

Fig. 1 The oral and skin manifestations of erythema multiforme

systemic treatment required.

Erythema multiforme[3] is an immunological reaction to a number of causes such as viral infections (especially herpes simplex) and drugs. The rash can assume several forms, but classically appears as 'target lesions' with a central bulla surrounded by concentric rings of erythema (*Fig. 1*). The condition tends to predominantly affect adolescent males with recurrent episodes often diminishing in severity with increasing age. The most severe form involves the eyes, mouth and genitalia (Stevens-Johnson syndrome). The disease is self-limiting and the use of systemic steroids is controversial.

Dermatitis herpetiformis is a rare blistering disorder in which IgA antibody is directed against the skin causing widespread, often small vesicles that are extremely itchy. The condition is often associated with coeliac disease but oral involvement is unusual. It usually responds well to dapsone and for those with associated coeliac disease, a gluten free diet can be beneficial.

2. SKIN INFECTIONS

Infections of the skin are common and can be divided into those caused by bacteria, viruses, fungi and parasites.

Bacterial infections

Furuncle is a deep abscess of a hair follicle due to infection with *Staphylococcus aureus*. Precipitating factors include poor hygiene, stress and diabetes mellitus although many cases develop for no specific reason. Such patients often carry the causative strain of *Staphylococcus* in the nose, axillae and groin.

A **carbuncle** is a larger Staphylococcal abscess which discharges pus through several sinuses.

Impetigo is a superficial skin infection caused by *Staphylococcus aureus*, sometimes with Streptococci in addition. The lesions are golden crusted and can spread quite rapidly. The condition is contagious and as a result can pervade an institution such as a nursery. Sometimes it accompanies infestation with scabies or lice.

Cellulitis describes a deeper spreading Streptococcal infection that involves the subcutaneous tissues and can spread quite widely. **Erysipelas** is a form of cellulitis and is a superficial infection due to *Streptococcus pyogenes*. The lesion is a well defined area of tender, red and oedematous skin and is often associated with fever and malaise. Recurrent episodes of cellulitis are not uncommon.[4]

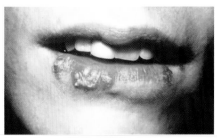

Fig. 2 Herpes simplex infection of the lip

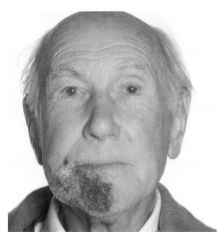

Fig. 3 Shingles - confined to the mandibular division of the trigeminal nerve

Viral infections

Verrucae (common warts) are common lesions that usually occur on the hands or soles (plantar warts) and are often self-limiting. Lesions can occur around the mouth, usually by auto-inoculation, particularly in thumb-suckers.

Herpes simplex infection is usually acquired from close contact with an infected individual during infancy. The primary infection involves painful vesicles/ulcers around the oral mucosa and gingivae. The condition is accompanied by fever, malaise and lymphadenopathy. It is usually self-limiting. In a number of cases the primary infection is sub-clinical, although once infected the virus remains for life and gives the potential for the development of secondary (recurrent) lesions.

Recurrent herpes infections may occur throughout life and are most commonly seen around the lips ('cold sores', *Fig. 2*). Attacks are often precipitated by febrile illness, local trauma, sunburn or menstruation. The lesion usually starts as a patch of localised painful erythema, in which develops a crop of clear vesicles that burst, crust and heal over a period of

ten days. Genital herpes follows the same pattern although the primary infection is usually acquired through sexual intercourse.

Herpes zoster infection, like herpes simplex, has a bimodal presentation with the primary condition usually being acquired in childhood as chickenpox (varicella zoster). The virus remains latent in the sensory root ganglia where it can become reactivated later in life causing shingles.

Shingles starts with pain, then erythema and vesicles in the distribution of a sensory nerve root. The preceding pain can be severe and occur up to two days before the development of the characteristic rash. Although any sensory nerve root distribution can be affected, it is most common on the trunk. The condition may involve any of the three branches of the trigeminal nerve and usually settles within two weeks, although it can leave pain in the affected region for several months afterwards (post-herpetic neuralgia). Lesions affecting the ophthalmic division of the trigeminal nerve may develop corneal damage and should be treated with an antiviral agent promptly to prevent long-term complications. Shingles affecting the mandibular division of the trigeminal nerve is shown in *Fig 3*.

The **Coxsackie group** of viruses can produce two infections of the oro-facial region; both are highly contagious but otherwise self-limiting. **Herpangina** produces characteristic painful lesions of the soft palate, accompanied by pyrexia and malaise. **Hand, foot and mouth disease** produces characteristic linear vesicles of the hands and feet, with shallow ulcers of the buccal mucosa. It is usually a mild self-limiting illness which often occurs as an epidemic in institutions.

Fungal infections

Numerous fungal infections can affect the skin but most have little effect on the oro-facial region. The most common yeast to affect the peri-oral region is the *Candida* species (usually albicans). This yeast is a common commensal in the mouth and being highly opportunistic, can cause a variety of intra-oral manifestations depending on local conditions such as poor denture hygiene or systemic disease. Spillage from the mouth can affect the adjacent skin, either alone or in combination with other opportunistic organisms such as *Staphylococcus aureus*, and give rise to **angular cheilitis**.

Angular cheilitis occurs as a result of saliva maceration at the corners of the mouth due to drooling or the presence of deep skin folds or ill-fitting dentures. Other factors that potentiate the development of secondary infection at this site are iron deficiency, diabetes mellitus or being immuno-compromised. In younger, dentate and otherwise fit individuals the condition is often solely an infection by *Staphylococcus aureus.*

In treating angular cheilitis it is important to assess for all possible contributing factors and to treat any accompanying intra-oral infection with an appropriate antifungal agent or the condition will recur.

3. DISORDERS OF HAIR

Hirsutism refers to growth of coarse hair in the 'male' pattern (especially in the beard area) occurring in a female. It is usually only a cosmetic defect but it can sometimes be a sign of over-production of androgen due to a tumour or hyperplasia of the ovary (polycystic ovaries) or adrenal gland. Affected individuals often have greasy skin and irregular periods.

Alopecia ('baldness') commonly happens in men with a family history of baldness and normal androgen levels. It rarely happens in women before the menopause and if it does occur in a young woman, it usually indicates an overproduction of androgens. Generally hair loss is more common with increasing age in both sexes.

Diffuse alopecia can occur in hypothyroidism, hypopituitarism, iron deficiency and (transiently) in pyrexial illness or childbirth. Some drugs, particularly cytotoxics, can also cause temporary hair loss. **Alopecia areata** is thought to be an autoimmune disorder resulting in patchy hair loss. Most cases recover spontaneously, but some progress to total hair loss, including the eyelashes and body hair (alopecia universalis).

4. DISORDERS OF PIGMENTATION

Malignant melanoma is considered in chapter 13.

Hyperpigmentation

The most common pigment in the skin is melanin produced by dendritic cells in the basal layer – melanocytes. All races have a similar number of melanocytes but those races with a darker skin have more active melanocytes. In general, melanin is protective against ultraviolet light and production of melanin occurs in direct response to exposure (sun tan). However, there are a number of conditions associated with an increase in pigmentation.

In adrenocortical deficiency as a result of destruction of the adrenal glands by either autoimmune (**Addison's disease**) or metastatic disease, overproduction of pituitary ACTH stimulates melanocytes to produce melanin. As a result the patient becomes pigmented and due to low or absent cortisol, has a poor tolerance to stress (such as in the dental surgery) and can develop steroid crisis (severe hypotension and collapse) without adequate steroid prophylaxis.

Certain drugs can result in increased pigmentation (eg busulphan) and a patchy hyperpigmentation can develop around the eyes and cheeks in pregnancy (melasma) or from the contraceptive pill.

Localised areas of hyperpigmentation can occur in old age (lentigenes) and peri-orally in **Peutz-Jeghers' syndrome**, an hereditary condition associated with intestinal polyps.

Hypopigmentation

Loss of pigment can be generalised, as in **albinism** (a congenital defect in melanin production), or localised such as in **vitiligo**. Vitiligo is probably an autoimmune disorder that destroys melanocytes. Although largely cosmetic, loss of pigment increases the risk of sun damage to the skin. Those affected should limit exposure and use appropriate sun block.

5. MISCELLANEOUS CONDITIONS – GENODERMATOSES

There is a genetic background in many skin disorders, but several are recognised as primarily genetic.

Ectodermal dysplasia is a rare, sex-linked recessive disorder characterised by sweat glands that fail to form (hypohidrosis) and scant hair (hypotrichosis) with absence of eyebrows and eyelashes. The importance of this condition in dentistry is that it is associated with hypodontia and abnormalities of tooth form.[5]

The term **epidermolysis bullosa** encompasses a group of rare bullous diseases affecting the skin and mucous membranes with various forms of inheritance. Vesicles and bullae form in response to mild or insignificant trauma and may lead to disabling scarring and deformity.

Neurofibromatosis type 1 (**von Recklinghausen's disease**) is an autosomal dominant condition characterised by multiple tumours of the nerve sheath (neurofibromas), in which sarcomatous change may develop, and patches of pigmented skin (café-au-lait spots).

Multiple basal cell naevi syndrome[6] (**Gorlin-Goltz syndrome**) is an autosomal dominant condition consisting of multiple basal cell carcinomas, odontogenic keratocysts and anomalies of the vertebrae, ribs and skull deformities, including calcification of the falx cerebri.

Tuberous sclerosis is an autosomal dominant trait characterised by epilepsy, learning disability and skin lesions in a butterfly pattern across the bridge of the nose, forehead and chin.

DENTAL MANAGEMENT OF PATIENTS WITH SKIN DISORDERS

Dental implications of various skin disorders likely to be seen in dental practice include direct involvement of the oral mucosa by a mucocutaneous disorder. In some circumstances, for example pemphigus, the oral lesions may precede the full blown condition and provide early diagnosis.

Some asymptomatic conditions in their early phase, such as basal cell carcinomas, commonly involve the facial skin and the dentist is in a good position to make the diagnosis and promote early referral. Some dermatological problems such as epidermolysis bullosa or systemic sclerosis may present specific problems in maintaining adequate oral hygiene and patients with these conditions require regular assistance. In such cases the wearing of dentures can prove extremely difficult and every effort to maintain the dentition should be taken.

A number of patients with dermatological conditions will be taking or have taken systemic steroids and may require steroid cover before any surgical intervention, such as extractions, to prevent steroid crisis. This is an area of controversy and some evidence suggests that the routine use of prophylactic steroids is unnecessary.[7] Many more patients will be using topical steroid medication, which could theoretically lead to adrenal suppression. However this appears not to be a problem and steroid cover for surgical dental procedures in this group is usually not required.

Many dermatological conditions are visible and cause considerable distress to those affected. Treatment by an understanding and knowledgeable practitioner can be of enormous reassurance to a sometimes emotionally vulnerable person.

From a dental perspective, patients affected with systemic sclerosis may be compromised by difficulty in accessing the oral cavity due to the taughtness of the circumoral skin. This can result in difficulty in maintaining adequate oral hygiene, a problem that can be exacerbated if the hands are affected to a degree where holding an oral hygiene aid such as a toothbrush becomes difficult.

Some skin conditions such as systemic lupus erythematosus are associated with a bleeding tendency caused by thrombocytopaenia and clotting defects (see below).

Considerations for treatment under local analgesia with or without sedation and general anaesthesia

As mentioned above, Addison's

disease is associated with hyperpigmentation and the lack of production of endogenous corticosteroids may lead to adrenal crisis. The use of prophylactic steroids is not universally advised for treatments on most patients receiving endogenous steroids (see below). The exception is the patient with Addison's disease, where steroid cover is still recommended.

Some of the systemic conditions such as systemic lupus erythematosus are associated with prolonged bleeding as a result of both thrombocytopaenia and a coagulation deficit as mentioned above. A careful history is required to see if the patient has any haemorrhagic problem and pre-surgical screening for platelet numbers and clotting studies may be required.

In cases of C1 esterase deficiency, supplementation before dental treatment may be provided to prevent the development of angio-oedema.

Dentists and their assistants may become sensitised to rubber gloves, medicaments or chemicals such as acrylic monomer resins producing a type IV (delayed) hypersensitivity reaction. Such hypersensitivity usually causes hand eczema, but aerosols can lead to facial eczema. Patch testing the skin (usually on the back) to a range of possible sensitisers for 48 hours is the usual way of identifying the cause. Treatment, like that for irritant eczema, is avoidance of the cause or the use of a barrier (eg hypo-allergenic gloves). It should be remembered with hypersensitivity reactions, however, that subsequent contact will lead to an exacerbated response and should be avoided at all costs. Acute flare-ups can be treated by a topical steroid cream or ointment.

IMPACT OF DRUGS

A number of different drugs are used in the management of skin disorders and an understanding of the impact of these on dental treatment is merited.

Corticosteroids

As mentioned above, the use of supplementary steroids is no longer considered essential for most patients

taking these drugs. Monitoring of the blood pressure is recommended during treatment and if the diastolic pressure drops by more than 25% then an intravenous injection of 100-200 mg hydrocortisone is required.

Patients taking long-term steroid therapy may be more susceptible to infections such as Candida and any acute infection should be treated without delay.

The use of non steroidal anti inflammatory drugs is not recommended in patients taking corticosteroids on a long-term basis as such a combination can lead to gastro-intestinal ulceration.

Antimicrobial drugs

Long-term tetracycline use, if it coincides with dental development, can lead to staining of the teeth. Tetracycline may also be a cause of lichenoid lesions intra-orally. This drug can reduce the efficacy of other antibacterials such as penicillin. Tetracycline is commonly used in the treatment of acne vularis.

Immunosuppressant drugs

A number of immunosuppressant drugs such as ciclosporin, tacrolimus and methotrexate are used in the management of skin disorders. Patients on immunosuppressant therapy are more at risk of oral and peri-oral malignancies and any suspicious lesions should be biopsied on an urgent basis. Ciclosporin can produce gingival overgrowth.[8] Drugs that dentists prescribe can interact with immunosuppressants, for example non-steroidal anti-inflammatory drugs increase the toxicity of ciclosporin, methotrexate and tacrolimus and antifungal agents such as miconazole and ketoconazole reduce metabolism of ciclosporin and tacrolimus. Immunosuppressants may reduce platelet numbers leading to post-extraction bleeding; a reduction in white cell count may also increase the likelihood of post-operative infection. Full blood counts will inform the clinician if such sequelae are likely.

Dapsone

Dapsone can produce Stevens-Johnson syndrome leading to oral ulceration and crusting of the lips. This drug can reduce the red and white cell count leading to poor post-surgical healing.

Retinoids

Patients receiving retinoids may complain of dry lips.

CONCLUSION

With the similarities between skin and oral mucosa, it is hardly surprising that some dermatological conditions may have an oral component that occasionally may even precede other manifestations. Many patients may not appreciate this connection which can only be ascertained by careful history taking and where appropriate, examination.

In addition, many serious skin conditions such as malignant neoplasia frequently occur on the face, enabling the dental practitioner to facilitate early diagnosis and referral. It is an area where close co-operation between different professionals is beneficial.

1. Scully C, Mignogna M. Oral mucosal disease: pemphigus. *Br J Oral Maxillofac Surg* 2008; **46:** 272–277.
2. Scully C, Lo Muzio L. Oral mucosal diseases: mucous membrane pemphigoid. *Br J Oral Maxillofac Surg* 2008; **46:** 358–366.
3. Scully C, Bagan J. Oral mucosal diseases: erythema multiforme. *Br J Oral Maxillofac Surg* 2008; **46:** 90–95.
4. Morris A D. Cellulitis and erysipelas. Clinical Evidence Online 2008; pii: 1708. http://clinicalevidence.bmj.com/ceweb/index.jsp.
5. Crawford P J, Aldred M J, Clarke A. Clinical and radiographic dental findings in X linked hypohidrotic ectodermal dysplasia. *J Med Genet* 1991; **28:** 181–185.
6. Manfredi M, Vescovi P, Bonanini M, Porter S. Nevoid basal cell carcinoma syndrome: a review of the literature. *Int J Oral Maxillofac Surg* 2004; **33:** 117–124.
7. Thomason J M, Girdler N M, Kendall-Taylor P, Wastell H, Weddell A, Seymour R A. An investigation into the need for supplementary steroids in organ transplant patients undergoing gingival surgery. *J Clin Periodontol* 1999; **26:** 577–582.
8. Kataoka M, Kido J, Shinohara Y, Toshihiko Nagata T. Drug-induced gingival overgrowth – a review. *Bio Pharm Bull* 2005; **28:** 1817–1821.

Chapter 15
Psychiatry

S. Brown, M. Greenwood and J. G. Meechan

IN BRIEF

- Mental illness is a common problem and can present in many ways.
- Psychiatric problems may not always be relevant to a patient's dental management, but a little knowledge may avoid problems.
- It is important to presume all patients have capacity to consent unless proven otherwise.
- Mental illness may affect dental professionals and it is important to know how to access help.

There are a significant number of patients in society who have some form of psychiatric disorder. It is important that dental practitioners have an awareness of the more common psychiatric disorders and their potential implications as they are likely to encounter them in clinical practice.

INTRODUCTION

Mental illness is common, affecting up to one in four people in the UK at some time in their lives.[1] It is thus highly likely that a dentist will encounter psychiatric problems in their personal and/or professional lives.

Psychiatric problems may present to the dentist in a number of ways. The oral problem may be incidental or part of the psychiatric symptomatology. Pure dental anxiety may influence management. Thus it is important that dentists have some understanding of the basic concepts of psychiatry and the nature of psychiatric disorders.

The dentist may encounter mental health problems in relation to one of the following:

1. The underlying psychiatric condition, for example anxiety disorder, is exacerbated by the visit to the dentist, or creates problems in management
2. A psychiatric illness may be detected by the dentist, for example psychogenic pain, eating disorders, substance abuse and occasionally psychosis
3. Dental complications of psychiatric illness, for example pain syndromes, bruxism, poor oral hygiene
4. The illness may be unrelated to the dental attendance but some understanding may be useful to aid management, for example dementia, learning disability, or in relation to medication
5. The dental professional may be affected by a mental illness, most commonly alcohol problems, depression.

This chapter provides an overview of how psychiatric symptoms might present to the dentist with a brief description of some common psychiatric syndromes (*Table 1*). Consent with reference to the Mental Capacity Act (2005) is briefly discussed, concluding with how to access support and advice from psychiatric services when required.

Table 1 Psychiatric disorders relevant to dentistry
Dental anxiety
Dental phobia
Obsessive compulsive disorder
Hypochondriasis
Psychogenic pain – atypical facial pain, TMJ dysfunction, atypical odontalgia, oral dysaesthesia
Eating disorders – anorexia nervosa, bulimia nervosa
Drug and alcohol misuse
Schizophrenia
Depression
Bipolar disorder ('manic depression')

1. THE UNDERLYING PSYCHIATRIC CONDITION IS EXACERBATED BY A VISIT TO THE DENTIST, OR CREATES PROBLEMS IN THE CONSULTATION

Anxiety

Anxiety can be a normal response to perceived danger, activating the sympathetic nervous system in the performance enhancing response commonly known as 'fight or flight'. If anxiety becomes too intense, frequent or persistent and interferes with daily life, it may be considered pathological and part of an anxiety disorder.

Certain circumstances will induce a 'state' of anxiety in all of us. Some people are naturally more anxious than others, however, with a high level of 'trait' anxiety, and may be predisposed to anxiety disorders. Anxiety symptoms may be physical or psychological (*Table 2*) and may be so severe the individual attempts to avoid all possible triggers, potentially restricting their lifestyle significantly.

Of particular interest to the dentist is dental anxiety. Some estimates suggest up to 90% of people experience significant levels of anxiety before visiting the dentist, with 40% of adults delaying or completely avoiding visits because of anxiety. This may be highly specific amounting to **odontophobia**, or be a feature of **generalised anxiety disorder**. Anxious patients may not tolerate dental procedures without prior measures to reduce their anxiety and may find it difficult to pay attention to questions or advice, leading to difficulties in communication.

A recent study[2] reported that in addition to apprehension about injections, common fears were seeing, hearing and feeling the vibrations of a dental drill. Specific questionnaires such as the Corah anxiety scale[3,4] are available to assess anxiety. These are not employed by many British dentists but are more likely to be used by practitioners providing intravenous sedation.[5] Management of anxiety need not necessarily include medication, though anxiolytics such as benzodiazepines may be beneficial in the short-term. Non-medical interventions of benefit include cognitive behavioural therapy. Ideally steps should be taken to avoid the development of dental anxiety in the first instance, particularly for children. Simple measures aimed at making the dental consultation a pleasant experience may be invaluable, with judicious use of lighting and music and perhaps adjusting one's attire.

Paranoia

Meaning literally 'outside the mind', this term describes extreme suspiciousness or mistrust without reason. It may be a symptom of a number of disorders, including **paranoid schizophrenia**, **psychotic depression**, **mania** or **drug and alcohol misuse**. It may also be a feature of **dementia**,

Table 2 Symptoms of anxiety	
Psychological	**Physical**
Worry Sense of dread Irritability Poor concentration Restlessness	Gastrointestinal: dry mouth, nausea, swallowing difficulties, disturbance of bowel habit Cardiovascular/Respiratory: shortness of breath, chest pain, palpitations, tachycardia Neuromuscular: headache, light-headedness, weakness, 'jelly legs', tremor, muscle aches Other: sweating

Table 3 Core features of depression	
Core features of depression	**Additional features**
Depressed mood: most days for most of day for two weeks or more	Diurnal variation of mood Poor appetite and weight loss Sleep disturbance
Lack of energy (anergia)	Poor concentration
Loss of enjoyment (anhedonia)	Psychomotor retardation or agitation
Hopelessness and suicidal ideation	Feelings of guilt and worthlessness
Loss of libido	
Delusions and hallucinations if severe (guilt, worthlessness, poverty or disease)	

or simply a personality trait which may or may not be part of a personality disorder. In all these conditions paranoia may be associated with hallucinations in any modality, as well as changes in behaviour and cognitive function.

A paranoid patient may, like a dental phobic, avoid the dentist altogether. Alternatively paranoia may lead to mistrust of the dentist's advice, complaints against the dentist, or seeking repeated consultations with different practitioners.

Depression

A lowering of mood may be a feature of many illnesses, or a side-effect of many common medications (eg Beta blockers). When severe enough to affect daily life and associated with symptoms such as disturbance of sleep, appetite and reduced enjoyment of usual activities, it may be part of a syndrome of clinical depression (*Table 3*). Depressive illness is very common, affecting up to 10% of men and 20% of women at some point in their lives.

The dentist may find such patients slow to answer questions, make decisions or grasp advice given and might

easily feel frustrated with their negativity or avoidance of eye contact. They may also have lower tolerance for pain or discomfort associated with dental conditions or treatment.

Disinhibition

This may be seen as part of a manic episode of bipolar disorder, or in patients with dementia or learning disability.

Bipolar affective disorder (manic depression) is characterised by discrete episodes of elevated mood (mania, or less severe hypomania) interspersed with episodes of either normal mood or periods of depressed mood. In an episode of elated mood, a patient may seem disinhibited either socially or sexually. They may be over-talkative, elated and excitable or agitated and at times dress or behave inappropriately. Concentration may be poor and patients may be unreliable historians. Although this is most likely to occur in the manic phase of bipolar disorder, alcohol, illicit drugs and occasionally prescribed medication such as steroids can cause a similar picture. Such a presentation could render dental intervention impossible during a particular visit, but is most likely to make the dentist uncomfortable; a chaperone is thus advisable at all times in the interests of both dentist and patient.

Hyperactivity

Extreme restlessness may be a side-effect of certain psychiatric drugs or a feature of stimulant drug use. Hyperactivity is most likely to be seen in children with attention deficit hyperactivity disorder (ADHD) and its variants. It may be particularly difficult to examine an overactive child and the environment of the dental surgery may prove hazardous. As with all children's consultations, if an examination is essential it may be useful to try to simplify the environment as much as possible in advance. Simple calming measures such as softer lighting and music, or projecting something to capture the child's attention on the ceiling may prove useful.

2. THE DENTIST MAY DETECT A PSYCHIATRIC ILLNESS

Some psychiatric disorders have significant dental signs and symptoms and may thus be noted for the first time in a dental consultation. This includes eating disorders, pain syndromes, use of certain illicit drugs and occasionally psychosis.

Eating disorders

Induced vomiting may be a feature of either **anorexia nervosa** or **bulimia nervosa**, leading to some specific signs pertinent to the dentist. Erosion of the dental enamel, especially on the palatal surfaces, may be caused by exposure to gastric acid in vomiting. This may be associated with callusing on the dorsum of the fingers (Russell's sign). In addition to affecting the dental hard tissues, eating disorders may be the cause of mucosal lesions such as erythema, periodontitis and salivary hypofunction.[6] As well as symptoms of malnutrition and vitamin deficiency there may be profound disturbances of electrolytes, particularly potassium, which can lead to fatal arrhythmias.

Pain syndromes

Up to 50% of psychogenic pain is experienced as occurring in the head. There are four major recognised syndromes: **atypical facial pain**, **temporomandibular joint dysfunction syndrome (TMD)** (facial arthromyalgia), **atypical odontalgia** and **oral dysaesthesia**. It can be difficult to distinguish between true pain of dental origin, for which a dental intervention may be appropriate, and psychogenic pain, particularly as the experience for the patient is as for real pain. Certain clues in the history may suggest a psychological origin, however, and these are summarised in *Table 4*.

Hypochondriasis

Occasionally the dentist may see a patient convinced of the presence of an underlying disease, despite an absence of physical signs or positive investigations. Multiple minor symptoms may be presented as evidence and these should be taken seriously, with relevant examination and investigations undertaken to exclude physical disease. If hypochondriasis is suspected, however, it is advisable to seek psychiatric help at an early stage, as prolonged investigations and repeated assessments will reinforce the illness beliefs and may in fact exacerbate the condition.

Table 4 Features suggestive of psychogenic pain
Inconsistency with known anatomical landmarks/nerve distribution
Bilateral
Continuous with little fluctuation
May prevent falling asleep but does not wake the patient up
History of repeated negative investigations
Analgesia has a very limited effect
Association with emotional factors
Nature of the pain may have a symbolic significance for the patient

Substance misuse

It is not only one's patients who are at risk of substance misuse – drug and alcohol problems are high among medical and dental professionals.[7] It is therefore worth being alert to the signs of problematic substance use which, untreated, can be devastating on a personal, social and professional level.

Misuse of drugs can cause many oro-dental manifestations and interfere with dental management.[8] A few examples are given here.

Dental consequences of misuse of the stimulant **methamphetamine** may include xerostomia, bruxism (which can lead to TMD), self-neglect and a rapidly deteriorating, advanced

Table 5 Potential drug interactions	
Drug type	**Interactions**
Antidepressants: Tricyclics (amitriptyline, clomipramine, imipramine, trimipramine, lofepramine)	Local anaesthetic: sympathomimetics (eg adrenaline) → hypertension and arrhythmias - not a contraindication to adrenaline but dose reduction is advised General anaesthetic (GA) → increased risk of cardiac arrhythmias and hypotension
MAOIs (monoamine-oxidase inhibitors, eg phenelzine)	GA → hypertension and arrhythmias Risk of hypertensive crisis – MAOI should be stopped two weeks before anaesthetic
Mood stabilisers: Lithium	Antibiotics, particularly metronidazole, may cause lithium toxicity NSAIDS, eg ibuprofen, diclofenac may cause lithium toxicity GA → enhanced hypotensive effect
Antipsychotics	Antibiotics Erythromycin → increased risk of convulsions with clozapine
Dementia drugs	Ketamine → toxic combination with memantine
ADHD drugs	GA → hypertension with methylphenidate

state of dental decay known as 'meth mouth'.[9]

Cocaine use can cause problems that may present to the dentist in the absence of overt dental pathology. Pain in the teeth and gums is a recognised feature of cocaine abuse and may be due to teeth grinding and jaw-clenching. The localised vasoconstriction produced by cocaine can cause gingival necrosis if this area is used by abusers to test the 'quality' of the drug.

Benzodiazepine withdrawal may cause a characteristic syndrome of paraesthesia, hypersensitivity and pain in the teeth or jaw in almost 50% of patients who try to stop or reduce these drugs, making a reduction in long-term use problematic. Similar problems may occur with **opiate** withdrawal.

Psychosis – (hallucinations and delusions)

Sometimes paranoia may take the form of a delusion – a fixed belief that persists despite evidence to the contrary and is at odds with the individual's culture, religion and circumstances. This may occur in psychotic depression or schizophrenia as well as mania or drug use.

An example of relevance to the dentist might be a patient complaining of pain or requesting an extraction in the belief that a transmitter has been implanted in a tooth.

3. DENTAL COMPLICATIONS OF PSYCHIATRIC ILLNESS

Oral dystonias, drooling and bruxism may be the extrapyramidal side-effects of a number of drugs used to treat psychiatric illness, primarily the older (but still used) 'typical' antipsychotics such as haloperidol, chlorpromazine, and most slow-release 'depot' medications. These, and the drugs commonly used to counter such side-effects, also have anticholinergic properties and may cause a dry mouth. Potential interactions with psychiatric drugs are summarised in *Table 5*.

Poor oral hygiene and general self-care may occur in chronic mental illness, resulting in advanced dental

Table 6 CAGE questionnaire	
C:	Have you ever felt you should Cut down the amount you drink?
A:	Are you Annoyed if people comment upon the amount you are drinking?
G:	Do you ever feel Guilty about the amount you are drinking
E:	Have you ever had a drink early in the morning as an 'Eye-opener'?

Table 7 Mental state examination	
Appearance and behaviour	How are they dressed? Are they clean? Shaven? Well-groomed, or dishevelled and unkempt or flamboyantly or scantily dressed for the weather? Still in their pyjamas or slippers? Do they seem withdrawn or slowed down? Overactive or intrusive? Jumpy or on-edge? Are they aggressive? Are there any notable mannerisms or unusual movements?
Speech	Fast or slow, quiet or loud, monotonous, repetitive, slurred or stuttering?
Thoughts	Form – are they in an ordered flow, or disordered, fragmented and disconnected? Content – is there a particular preoccupation? Are there unusual beliefs which are held firmly and may not be based in reality (delusions)?
Mood	Objective (practitioner's view) and subjective (the patient's view) – elated, depressed, neither? Reactivity – is there an emotional response to sad or funny material? Is the response as would be expected?
Abnormal sensory experiences	Hallucinations – do they seem to be responding to sensory stimuli which cannot be detected? Or are there misperceptions of stimuli?
Cognitive functioning	Orientation – do they know where they are in time and place and who they are? Memory – can they recall how they got there? Can they recall their last appointment, or what advice they received? Concentration – are they following discussion? Where is their attention? Poor concentration may make memory seem impaired.
Insight	Do they recognise there is a problem? Do they understand it? Are they willing to receive help or treatment?

caries or infection with late presentation to the dentist. This may also occur in dementia and people with learning disabilities, occasionally requiring multiple extractions or total dental clearance.

4. PSYCHIATRIC ILLNESS PRESENT BUT UNRELATED TO DENTAL PROBLEMS

In many cases the presence of psychiatric illness may be of no relevance to dental management, particularly for routine work. Nonetheless it can be useful to have some understanding of certain conditions and in particular the drugs used to treat them.

Dementia

Dementia is defined as an acquired impairment of global cognitive function, which is generally progressive and largely irreversible. It is a disorder which is of relevance to most healthcare professionals. Alzheimer's disease is the most common cause of dementia, with a prevalence increasing significantly with age. Approximately 1% of 65-year-olds, 5% of 75-year-olds and 20% of 85-year-olds are affected.[10] Vascular dementia due to atherosclerosis is also common though there are also several other types of dementia.

The patient in the early stages of dementia may not seem cognitively impaired, but may struggle to take in new information and may therefore not follow the dentist's advice. In cases of more advanced dementia the disability will be obvious and it may be a challenge to persuade the patient to co-operate with a dental examination. In both cases dental pain or the presence of infection may significantly exacerbate any cognitive impairment or confusion and swift treatment can lead to dramatic improvements in function.

Learning disability

'Learning disability' is the term used to describe the presence of an intellectual deficit present from childhood.

It should be remembered that although a carer may seem to speak for patients with cognitive impairments, under the Mental Capacity Act (2005) all individuals over 16 years of age are presumed to have capacity unless proven otherwise. Consent should thus always be sought from the patient regardless of the apparent extent of their impairment.

5. THE DENTAL PROFESSIONAL MAY BE AFFECTED BY A MENTAL ILLNESS

Most common conditions have already been mentioned; depression (see above) and alcohol misuse are perhaps the most relevant in this scenario.

Alcohol

Alcohol abuse may be suspected if the individual smells of alcohol or has a tremor, which could be due to withdrawal. Attention should be paid to the time of day, as those with alcohol dependence may drink early in the morning to overcome withdrawal phenomena. The CAGE questionnaire (*Table 6*) is a simple and useful screening tool to detect alcohol dependency. Patients scoring 2 or more are highly likely to have alcohol problems but a negative CAGE response does not rule out alcohol misuse.

CAPACITY AND CONSENT

It is easy to assume that patients suffering from significant psychiatric illnesses, dementia, learning disability or other impairments may not have the capacity to make their own decisions about treatment or to give consent; indeed dentists may at times find themselves under pressure from

relatives and carers to accept their decisions made on behalf of a patient.

The Mental Capacity Act (2005)[11] (introduced into practice in 2007) is an important piece of legislation designed to protect the rights of individuals to make their own decisions and provides guidelines to address this. It sets out guidance for decision-making on behalf of people who lack decision-making capacity and applies to all people aged 16 and over in England and Wales.

Decision-making capacity is considered to be task-specific, relevant only to a specific decision at a given time and should not be generalised to other situations and decisions.

There are five basic principles:
• **Autonomy:** presumption of capacity. People are presumed to have capacity until proven otherwise
• Decision-making capacity must be maximised by all practicable means
• An individual has the right to make an unwise decision
• **Best interests:** decisions or acts taken on behalf of a person who is found to lack capacity must be taken in their best interests
• **Least restrictive:** the least restrictive decision or action should be taken, where an individual is found to lack decision-making capacity.

Capacity should be assessed by the person who is proposing treatment and seeking consent, using a standard two part question:
1. Is there an impairment of, or a disturbance in the functioning of, the mind or brain?
2. If so, does its presence impair the person's ability to make a particular decision?

A four-stage test adapted from common law must then be applied, looking at the decision-making process itself:

'A person is unable to make a decision for himself if he/she is unable—
(a) To understand the information relevant to the decision
(b) To retain that information (for at

least long enough to make the decision)
(c) To use or weigh that information as part of the process of making the decision, or
(d) To communicate his/her decision (whether by talking, using sign language or any other means).'

Relevant information should be provided in a manner appropriate to the needs of the patient, involving an interpreter where necessary, and the patient should be similarly aided in communicating his/her decision. There is also a requirement to attempt to determine whether a lasting power of attorney (LPA) exists, appointing someone to act on their behalf in relation to health and welfare decisions.

If an individual is found to be lacking the capacity to make a particular decision, there are two possible courses of action – either to defer treatment and reassess, or to act in 'best interests'. 'Best interests' must be determined on an individual basis, taking into account all possible sources of information and may require the involvement of an independent mental capacity advocate (IMCA). The Act contains guidance for doing this.

Further information is contained within the Mental Capacity Act and its Code of Practice, and guidance is freely available for healthcare professionals through organisations such as the British Medical Association.[12]

Table 8 High risk characteristics for suicide
Male > Female
Age > 40 years (increasing in young men)
Evidence of planning
Social classes I and V
Certain occupations: dentists, doctors, vets, lawyers
Unemployed
Living alone
Not married
Loss events: relationships, housing, finance

WHAT TO DO WHEN PROBLEMS ARISE

There are no hard and fast rules about who should or should not be referred for further assessment. A number of scenarios may arise in dental practice:

• New presentation of psychiatric illness – such patients should be encouraged to speak to their general medical practitioner (GMP) about whatever symptoms have been noticed. It is not necessary to suggest it may be due to psychiatric illness

• Deterioration of existing illness – these patients should be asked to speak to their GMP or existing psychiatric services

• Overt suicidal ideation (either as new or altered presentation) – such patients should be advised to speak to their GMP or go to A&E, or the on-call psychiatric services or police should be contacted directly

• Patient presenting an immediate danger to others – call the police

• You or a colleague need help – a GMP or A&E should be able to help, or contact the confidential Dentists' Health Support Programme.

PSYCHIATRIC ASSESSMENT

As with all assessments, the psychiatric history focuses on the presenting complaint, followed by detailed contextual information including previous psychiatric problems, physical health problems, medication and a detailed developmental, personal and social history. A physical examination remains relevant and can reveal many clues as to the source of the psychiatric symptoms (eg hyper- or hypothyroidism, needle-tracks from injection of illicit drugs, neurological abnormalities). The main difference in a psychiatric assessment is the mental state examination, which requires careful observation of the patient and provides valuable clues as to which diagnosis should be reached (*Table 7*), and the risk assessment.

Risk assessment

Contrary to what the media would have us believe, patients with psychiatric illness are rarely a risk to others. Around 5% of all homicides are committed by people with a diagnosis of schizophrenia. Drug or alcohol abuse, however, are thought to contribute to over half of all murders. Far more likely is the risk to self, either through self-neglect due to illness, self-harm or suicide. While the best predictor of future behaviour is past behaviour, there are also a number of risk factors recognised to increase the likelihood of suicide, not all of which may be modified. Some of these are summarised in *Table 8*.

Along with doctors and lawyers, dentists are recognised as a group of professionals at a high risk of mental health problems including drug and alcohol misuse and suicide. Recognising and understanding problems in oneself or in colleagues may be just as important as recognising and understanding them in our patients.

CONCLUSION

Psychiatric problems are common and are likely to be encountered in routine dental practice. Many disorders have common symptoms that may be managed using the same general guiding principles, aiming to alleviate distress and anxiety, and respecting the individual's autonomy. Communication with carers may be important, as well as liaising with the patient's GMP or psychiatric services when necessary.

1. Crisp A H (ed). Every family in the land. London: Royal Society of Medicine Press, 2005.
2. Boyle C A, Newton T, Milgrom P. Who is referred for sedation for dentistry and why? *Br Dent J* 2009; **206:** E12.
3. Corah N L. Development of a dental anxiety scale. *J Dent Res* 1969; **48:** 596.
4. Corah N L, Gale E N, Illig S J. Assessment of a dental anxiety scale. *J Am Dent Assoc* 1978; **97:** 816–819.
5. Dailey Y M, Humphris G M, Lennon M A. Dental anxiety: the use of dental anxiety questionnaires: a survey of UK dental practitioners. *Br Dent J* 2001; **190:** 450–453.
6. Russo L L, Campisi G, Di Fede O, Panzarella V, Muzio L L. Oral manifestations of eating disorders: a critical review. *Oral Dis* 2008; **14:** 479–484.
7. Newbury-Birch D, Lowry R J, Kamali F. The changing patterns of drinking, illicit drug use, stress, anxiety and depression in dental students in a UK dental school: a longitudinal study. *Br Dent J* 2002; **192:** 646–649.
8. Meechan J G. Drug abuse and dentistry. *Dent Update* 1999; **26:** 182-190.
9. McGrath C, Chan B. Oral health sensations associated with illicit drug abuse. *Br Dent J* 2005; **198:** 159–162.
10. Knapp M, Prince M, Albanese E et al. Dementia UK. The full report. London: The Alzheimer's Society, 2007.
11. Office of Public Sector Information. The Mental Capacity Act 2005. Available online at http://www.opsi.gov.uk/acts/acts2005/20050009.htm.
12. BMA Ethics. The Mental Capacity Act 2005. Guidance for health professionals. London: British Medical Association, 2009. http://www.bma.org.uk/ethics/consent_and_capacity/mencapact05.jsp.

Chapter 16
Cancer, radiotherapy and chemotherapy

P. J. Thomson, M. Greenwood and J. G. Meechan

IN BRIEF

- Dentists will encounter patients with various types of cancer who require dental care.
- Patients may be at various stages of cancer treatment but the dentist may be involved at any stage.
- A working knowledge of the potential effects of cancer and its treatment is essential for safe practice.

Dental practitioners will encounter patients who have been affected by cancer or who are current cancer patients. Dentists play an important role in the overall healthcare of such patients, particularly in those with head and neck malignancy. This chapter gives an overview of the impact of cancer and its treatment on dental mangement.

INTRODUCTION

Cancer is the term applied to malignant tumours and is essentially a genetic disease caused by somatic mutation. The multi-stage theory of carcinogenesis suggests that individual cancers arise from several sequential mutations in cellular DNA. There is a close correlation between cancer incidence and increased age, reflecting the time required to accumulate the critical number of genetic abnormalities needed for malignant change.

Improvement in cancer treatment outcomes means that in modern clinical practice, a general dental practitioner will have to advise and treat many patients requiring oral healthcare with malignancies at various stages of the disease.

POINTS IN THE HISTORY

As a consequence of their malignancy, patients with cancer may suffer from a number of general physical, medical and emotional problems. It is important that dental practitioners have an understanding not only of the effects of malignant disease on their patient, but also of the specific problems resulting from cancer treatments (*Table 1*). While the range, symptomatology and diagnosis of malignant neoplasms presenting in the head and neck region will be well known to dentists (*Table 2*), the effects of cancer treatment may not be and it is often this area that leads to confusion and compromised dental care.

In general, malignant neoplasms are treated using one, or some combination of the following treatment modalities:
- Surgery
- Radiotherapy
- Chemotherapy.

The patient may give a history of having experienced such treatment, may be undergoing it or waiting for it. The selection, timing and prescription of these anticancer treatments is now the remit of highly specialised multidisciplinary oncology teams and varies considerably depending upon tumour type and site. While the principles of surgical access, tumour resection with wide margins and tissue reconstruction are familiar to dentists, particularly in relation to

Table 1 General complications of cancer
Cachexia and wasting
Anaemia and infection
Nutritional deficiencies
Cutaneous manifestations
Endocrine disorders
Rare manifestations

Table 2 Orofacial manifestations of cancer
Primary tumours in orofacial tissues
Oral squamous cell carcinoma
Salivary adenocarcinoma
Metastases in jaws or oral soft tissues
From breast, lung and prostate primaries
Effects of tumour metabolites
Facial flushing
Pigmentations
Amyloidosis
Oral erosions
Functional disturbances
Purpura
Bleeding
Infections
Anaemia

Table 3 Chemotherapy drugs and regimens		
Drug classification	**Examples**	
Alkylating agents	Busulphan Chlorambucil Cyclophosphamide	
Cytotoxic antibiotics	Bleomycin Doxorubicin	
Antimetabolites	Fluorouracil Methotrexate	
Vinca alkaloids	Vinblastine Vincristine	
Platinum compounds	Cisplatin	
Treatment regimen	**Administration**	**Aim**
Induction	Before other treatments	Reduce tumour size
Sandwich	Between treatments	Reduce risk of metastases
Adjuvant	After treatment	Improve disease-free survival
Concurrent	With other treatments	Sensitise tumour cells
Palliative	After other treatments	Shrink residual tumours Pain relief

Table 4 Oral complications of cancer therapy
Radiotherapy
Mucositis/ulceration
Radiation caries/dental hypersensitivity/periodontal disease
Xerostomia/loss of taste
Dysphagia
Candidosis
Osteoradionecrosis
Trismus
Craniofacial defects (children)
Chemotherapy
Mucositis/ulceration/lip cracking
Infections
Bleeding
Orofacial pain

orofacial cancers, the mechanism of action, efficacy and side-effects of radiotherapy and chemotherapy are often less well understood.

A patient may give a history of planned or previous radiotherapy. It is possible, but more unlikely, that they are undergoing radiotherapy at the time of attendance for dental treatment. Radiotherapy refers to the therapeutic application of localised ionising radiation (X-rays, beta rays or gamma rays) to destroy malignant cells. Cells exposed to radiation form free radicals in their intracellular water and, as a result of DNA damage, undergo death when stimulated to divide. Radiotherapy is thus particularly effective against rapidly proliferating tumour cells which are killed more efficiently than slowly growing or normal cells. While this is a considerable advantage in cancer treatment, it does not spare normal cells with high replication rates such as epithelium of skin and mucous membranes or highly specialised cells in neurological tissue, salivary gland secretory tissue or osteoblasts in bone which, when damaged, are unable to repair themselves. Other types of radiation may also be employed; for example, radioactive iodine (given orally or by intravenous injection) can be used to treat thyroid cancers. Such treatment can affect the function of the salivary glands.[1]

Patients may reveal a history of chemotherapy or be awaiting or undergoing this modality of treatment. The use of chemotherapeutic agents (anticancer drugs) is most often employed systemically in the treatment of widespread malignancies such as leukaemia or lymphoma, although more recent recognition of early systemic spread of solid tumours such as breast cancer and even head and neck malignancy has resulted in greater use of chemotherapy in modern treatment protocols. Chemotherapy agents (Table 3) target actively dividing cells to eliminate tumours while allowing normal cells to recover and repair. Drugs are usually administered in high doses intermittently and often in combination to achieve synergy and overcome resistance. Newer head and neck regimens utilise chemotherapy agents administered as radiosensitisers before radiotherapy to increase treatment efficacy but this may also enhance treatment side-effects.

EXAMINATION

The patient with cancer may look relatively well or may be cachectic. The term cachexia refers to a profound and marked state of constitutional disorder, general ill health and malnutrition. The signs and symptoms of oral cancer are well covered in relevant texts and therefore will not be covered further here.

The orofacial region contains one of the highest concentrations of specialised tissues and sensory organs in the body and it is hardly surprising that the effects of cancer treatment are particularly severe here. The cellular damage effects of radiotherapy and chemotherapy produce similar effects on oral tissues, although more widespread and systemic complications occur following chemotherapy. Table 4 lists the oral complications of radiotherapy and chemotherapy which may be seen on examination.

Mucositis is a particularly distressing condition arising from damage to the oral mucosal lining. It presents as widespread oral erythema, pain, ulceration and bleeding. It may arise during localised head and neck radiotherapy or as a consequence of systemic chemotherapy. Although an acute and usually relatively short-lived problem, it can significantly impair quality of life and prevent oral dietary intake leading to hospitalisation. If it is particularly severe it may cause interruption to therapeutic regimens and can act as a portal for septicaemia.

Xerostomia is responsible for the most common and long-standing problems following orofacial radiotherapy. Salivary gland function rarely recovers following secretory cell damage and while newer computerised radiotherapy techniques help to spare full salivary gland irradiation, it remains difficult to avoid gland damage. As mentioned above, salivary gland damage may also occur secondary to the use of radioactive iodine for the destruction of thyroid tumours.

Permanent mouth dryness, glutinous sputum in the posterior oral cavity and pharynx, and reduction of or altered taste, together with fragile and sensitive oral mucosa, are significant post-radiotherapy sequelae impairing a patient's quality of life. Xerostomia also increases the risk of rapidly destructive dental caries ('radiation caries') and advanced periodontal disease. Artificial saliva preparations including saliva sprays, replacement gels or pastilles may be helpful. Oral administration of pilocarpine may help to increase flow in patients with residual salivary gland function.

Infections are common due to immunosuppression, especially candidal and herpetic types. Appropriate use of antifungal agents such as miconazole or systemic fluconazole may be necessary to treat severe oral candidosis.

The lesions of osteoradionecrosis, as shown in *Fig. 1* (non-vital bone secondary to radiotherapy), or osteonecrosis as in *Fig. 2* (non-vital bone secondary to bisphosphonate treatment) may be evident and should be managed as described in the next section.

DENTAL MANAGEMENT OF HEAD AND NECK CANCER PATIENTS

The important management principles for patients undergoing radiotherapy for head and neck malignancy are

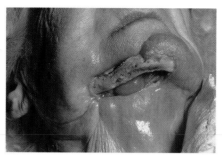

Fig. 1 A patient with osteoradionecrosis. The overlying skin has broken down due to its poor blood supply

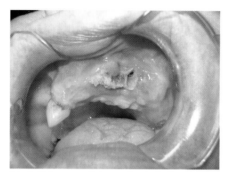

Fig. 2 Osteonecrosis in a patient who has been prescribed bisphosphonates and has had dental extractions in this area

summarised in *Table 5*. The general dental practitioner has an important role in management. It is important that the patient is rendered dentally fit before the commencement of radiotherapy treatment. This also applies to patients about to receive chemotherapy. The principles of management are summarised in *Table 6*.

The importance of general dental care and oral hygiene, especially for head and neck cancer patients, cannot be emphasised too strongly. A comprehensive dental assessment and proactive preventive treatment plan is mandatory before definitive head and neck cancer treatment. While this is often led by specialist restorative dentists working in multidisciplinary oncology teams, the role of the general dental practitioner remains central.

Patients undergoing radiotherapy for orofacial cancers need dental input to minimise radiation caries, the need for post-radiotherapy dental extractions and to reduce the risk of osteoradionecrosis. Extractions are advised for grossly carious, non-vital, periodontally involved teeth or retained roots and their removal

Table 5 Management of patients receiving head and neck radiotherapy
Before radiotherapy
Oral hygiene/preventive and restorative dentistry
Risk/benefits of retaining teeth
Dental extractions
During radiotherapy
Discourage smoking and alcohol
Eliminate infections: antibiotics/antifungals/antivirals
Relieve mucositis
Saliva substitutes
TMJ physiotherapy for trismus
After radiotherapy
Oral hygiene/preventive dentistry
Specialist OMFS for dental extractions/oral surgery
Topical fluorides
Avoidance of mucosal trauma
Saliva substitutes

Table 6 Management of patients receiving chemotherapy
Before chemotherapy
Oral/dental assessment
Oral hygiene/preventive dentistry
During chemotherapy
Folic acid to reduce ulceration
Ice to cool oral mucosa
Chlorhexidine mouthwashes
Eliminate infections: antibiotics/antifungals/antivirals
After chemotherapy
Oral hygiene/preventive dentistry
Risk of anaemia/bleeding/infection

should be performed carefully before radiotherapy starts to ensure rapid healing.

Osteoradionecrosis arises due to the death of irradiated and lethally damaged bone cells stimulated to divide following traumatic stimuli such as dental extractions or localised infection (*Fig. 1*). Diminished vascularity of the periosteum also exists as a result of late radiation effects on endothelial lining cells, which is particularly pertinent for the dense and less vascular mandibular bone. The radionecrotic process usually starts as ulceration of the alveolar mucosa with brownish dead bone exposed at the base. Pathological fractures may occur in weakened bone and secondary infection leads to severe discomfort, trismus, foetor oris and general malaise. Radiographically, the earliest changes are a 'moth-eaten' appearance of the bone, followed by sequestration.

Treatment should be predominantly conservative, with long-term antibiotic and topical antiseptic therapy and careful local removal of sequestra when necessary. Hyperbaric oxygen and ultrasound therapy to increase tissue blood flow and oxygenation have also been recommended[2] and are used as a treatment modality in the UK.[3]

Osteonecrosis is a recently recognised complication of bisphosphonate treatment[4] (*Fig. 2*). This condition is defined as exposed bone in the maxillofacial region for longer than eight weeks in the absence of radiotherapy but in a patient using bisphosphonates. It is diagnosed clinically but local malignancy must be excluded.[5] Bisphosphonates are a group of drugs, including alendronic acid, disodium etidronate and risedronate sodium, which are adsorbed onto hydroxyapatite crystals thus slowing their rate of growth and dissolution. They have been used in treatment of bony metastases, the hypercalcaemia of malignancy and the management of osteoporosis in post-menopausal women.

Dental extractions should be avoided wherever possible while patients are on bisphosphonate therapy to reduce the risk of necrosis. Established cases require analgesia, long-term antibiotic and topical antiseptic therapy, together with careful local debridement to remove limited bony sequestra similar to the management of osteoradionecrosis.[6] Risk factors that will increase the possibility of osteonecrosis developing include local infection, steroid use, trauma, chemotherapy and periodontal disease.

The mechanism by which bisphosphonates increase the risk of osteonecrosis is not fully understood. Trauma caused by dental extraction in the presence of impaired osteoclast function may cause inadequate clearance of necrotic debris. Local osteonecrosis may also occur due to secondary infection. It is also thought that bisphosphonates might have toxic effects on soft tissues around the extraction site and thereby impair the function of vascular and epithelial cells.[5]

Chemotherapy agents are inevitably highly toxic and risk important systemic effects such as infections and bleeding due to bone marrow involvement and resultant neutropaenia and thrombocytopaenia. It is important to liaise with an individual patient's oncologist to ensure dental or oral surgical treatments are timed to avoid periods of maximum bone marrow depression.

Management of established mucositis includes systemic analgesia, the use of intraoral ice and topical analgesics such as benzydamine hydrochloride or 2% lidocaine lollipops or mouthwash.

Subsequent to radiotherapy and chemotherapy, meticulous oral hygiene is essential, especially during treatment when the mouth is inflamed and sore. Dilute chlorhexidine mouthwashes, topical fluoride applications, saliva substitutes and active restorative care may all be needed to preserve the remaining dentition. Should teeth have to be extracted, this is best carried out in a specialist oral and maxillofacial surgery unit and it is essential that atraumatic techniques are used, with primary closure of oral mucosa together with antibiotic therapy until healing is complete. Similar considerations apply to patients taking bisphosphonates. The timing of extractions in patients undergoing chemotherapy is critical. This should be co-ordinated with the treating oncologist so that the ideal 'window of opportunity' is used.

EFFECTS OF DRUGS USED IN PATIENTS WITH ORAL MALIGNANCY ON DENTAL MANAGEMENT

As mentioned above, many drugs used in the management of malignant disease will affect white cell and platelet numbers. This means that bleeding and infection are risks of surgical dentistry such as extractions. A full blood count is needed to ensure that any extractions can be performed safely. Elective extractions should be carried out when the blood picture is normal, however emergency extractions may need to be performed. If the platelet count is less than 50×10^9 per litre then intra-oral surgery is contraindicated unless a platelet transfusion can be provided; if less than 100×10^9 per litre then sockets should be packed with a haemostatic agent such as Surgicel® and sutured. If the white cell count is less than 2.5×10^9 per litre then prophylactic antibiotics are recommended.

It was mentioned above that xerostomia and stomatitis are side-effects of radiotherapy. These can also be unwanted effects of some drugs used to treat malignancy. Thus excellent oral hygiene and caries prevention measures such as the use of fluoride are recommended. If dentures are ill-fitting these should be removed as they may worsen drug-induced mucositis.

Some of the drugs used to treat malignancies will interfere with medications dentists might prescribe. Examples include paracetamol and metronidazole, both of which increase the toxicity of busulphan by inhibiting metabolism and increasing plasma concentration of the cytotoxic drug. Similarly, erythromycin increases the toxicity of the chemotherapeutic drug vinblastine. The toxicity of methotrexate is increased with concomitant administration of non-steroidal anti-inflammatory drugs, penicillins and tetracyclines. These are just some examples of pertinent drug interactions. The dentist should consult a publication such as the *British National Formulary* or discuss with the patient's oncologist if there is any doubt about prescribing another medication.

Patients who have received treatment for childhood cancers may have dentofacial abnormalities as normal development may have been compromised. Problems such as poor root formation, enamel defects, prominent incremental lines in dentine and facial asymmetry may arise.[7,8]

CONCLUSIONS

Many patients with cancer will present to their dental practitioner requiring routine dental care or specific attention to oral complications resulting from malignancy or radiotherapy and chemotherapy treatments. It is imperative that dental practitioners make an appropriate assessment of the patient's general medical status (including nutrition, debilitation and haematology) before embarking upon dental care. Prevention is vital throughout to avoid worsening dental disease in patients with compromised general health.

1. Mandel S J, Mandel L. Radioactive iodine and the salivary glands. *Thyroid* 2003; **13:** 265–271.
2. Vudiniabola S, Pirone C, Williamson J, Goss A N. Hyperbaric oxygen in the therapeutic management of osteonecrosis of the facial bones. *Int J Oral Maxillofac Surg* 2000; **29:** 435–438.
3. Kanatas A N, Lowe D, Harrison J, Rogers S N. Survey of the use of hyperbaric oxygen by maxillofacial oncologists in the UK. *Br J Oral Maxillofac Surg* 2005; **43:** 219–225.
4. Hellstein J W, Marek C L. Bisphosphonate osteochemocrosis (bis-phossy jaw): is this phossy jaw of the 21st century? *J Oral Maxillofac Surg* 2005; **63:** 682–689.
5. Khan A. Osteonecrosis of the jaw and bisphosphonates. *BMJ* 2010; **340:** c246.
6. Migliorati C A, Casiglia J, Epstein J, Jacobsen P L, Siegel M A, Woo S B. Managing the care of patients with bisphosphonate-associated osteonecrosis: an American Academy of Oral Medicine position paper. *J Am Dent Assoc* 2005; **136:** 1658–1668.
7. Macleod R I, Welbury R R, Soames J V. Effects of cytotoxic chemotherapy on dental development. *J R Soc Med* 1987; **80:** 207–209.
8. Estilo C L, Huryn J M, Kraus D H et al. Effects of therapy on dentofacial development in long-term survivors of head and neck rhabdomyosarcoma: the Memorial Sloan Kettering cancer center experience. *J Pediatr Oncol* 2003; **25:** 215–222.